THE METBBLIC WAY

UNLOCKING OPTIMAL HEALTH: YOUR COMPREHENSIVE GUIDE TO METABOLIC WELLNESS

ZHAMEESHA LLC
ATLANTIS, FL (USA)

The METBBLIC Way
Unlocking Optimal Health:
Your Comprehensive Guide to Metabolic Wellness

Copyright © 2025 by Stuart Barry Malin

ISBN 978-1-951645-29-8
First Edition, Print on Demand
This version was most recently updated 2025-04-07

Published by Zhameesha LLC
Atlantis, Florida USA
https://www.zhameesha.com

This book is a work of compassion.

BISAC Subject Headings (www.bisg.org)
HEA048000   HEALTH & FITNESS / Diet & Nutrition / General
SEL000000   SELF-HELP / General
POL000000   POLITICAL SCIENCE / General

12 11 10 9 8 7 6 5 4 3 2 1

Welcome to **The METBBLIC Way**. This is our way of life and because we feel strongly that it has brought us health and well-being, we are inspired to share this with you!

At METBBLIC, we believe that vibrant health is not a luxury—it should be the norm. Yet, we live in a world where misinformation, industry-driven agendas, and misguided health policies have led many down a path of dependency, chronic illness, and confusion.

It's time to break free.

That's why we created **The METBBLIC Way**—a simple yet profound framework rooted in foundational truth, essential freedom, and personal responsibility. Inspired by the Hindi word *Samany*, meaning common and everyday, we envision a world where exceptional health isn't rare or difficult—it's the standard.

The METBBLIC Way cuts through the lies, noise, and disinformation exposing the truth about metabolism, food, and optimal living.

This booklet will introduce you to five core principles that will help you reclaim control over your health:

1. **Metabolic Truth** – Understanding what truly fuels energy, vitality, and longevity.
2. **Nutritional Freedom** – Breaking away from industry-driven misinformation and restrictive dogma.
3. **Personal Responsibility** – Owning your health choices and outcomes.

4. **Strategic Eating** – Learning how to nourish your body for peak performance.

5. **Longevity & Performance** – Thriving, not just surviving.

This isn't just another health guide—it's a call to action. Your health is in your hands. The choices you make today will shape your future. Are you ready to take control and live as if your life depends on it?

Welcome to the truth. Welcome to *The METBBLIC Way*.

Let's begin.

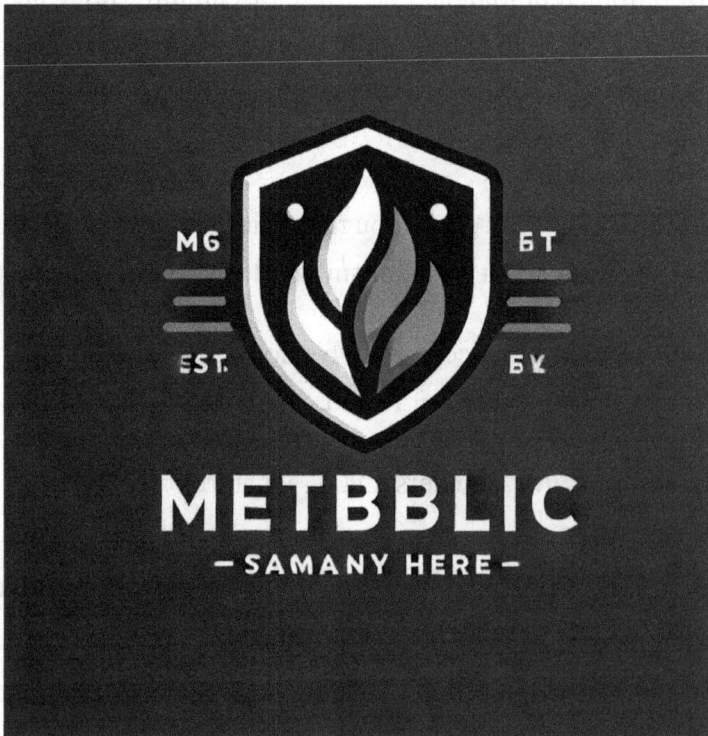

Contents

Welcome

Introduction & Background

Section 1 — Core Principles

The five core principles for metabolic wellness and vitality

Section 2 — Nutritional Freedom

Nutritional freedom requires breaking free from industry-driven myths

Section 3 — Fuel Your Body

How to fuel your body for strength, energy, and longevity

Section 4 - Personal Responsibility

The power of personal responsibility in reclaiming your health

Section 5 - Why This Is So

Thought Provoking Propositions About Why The System is Rigged Against You

Postmatter

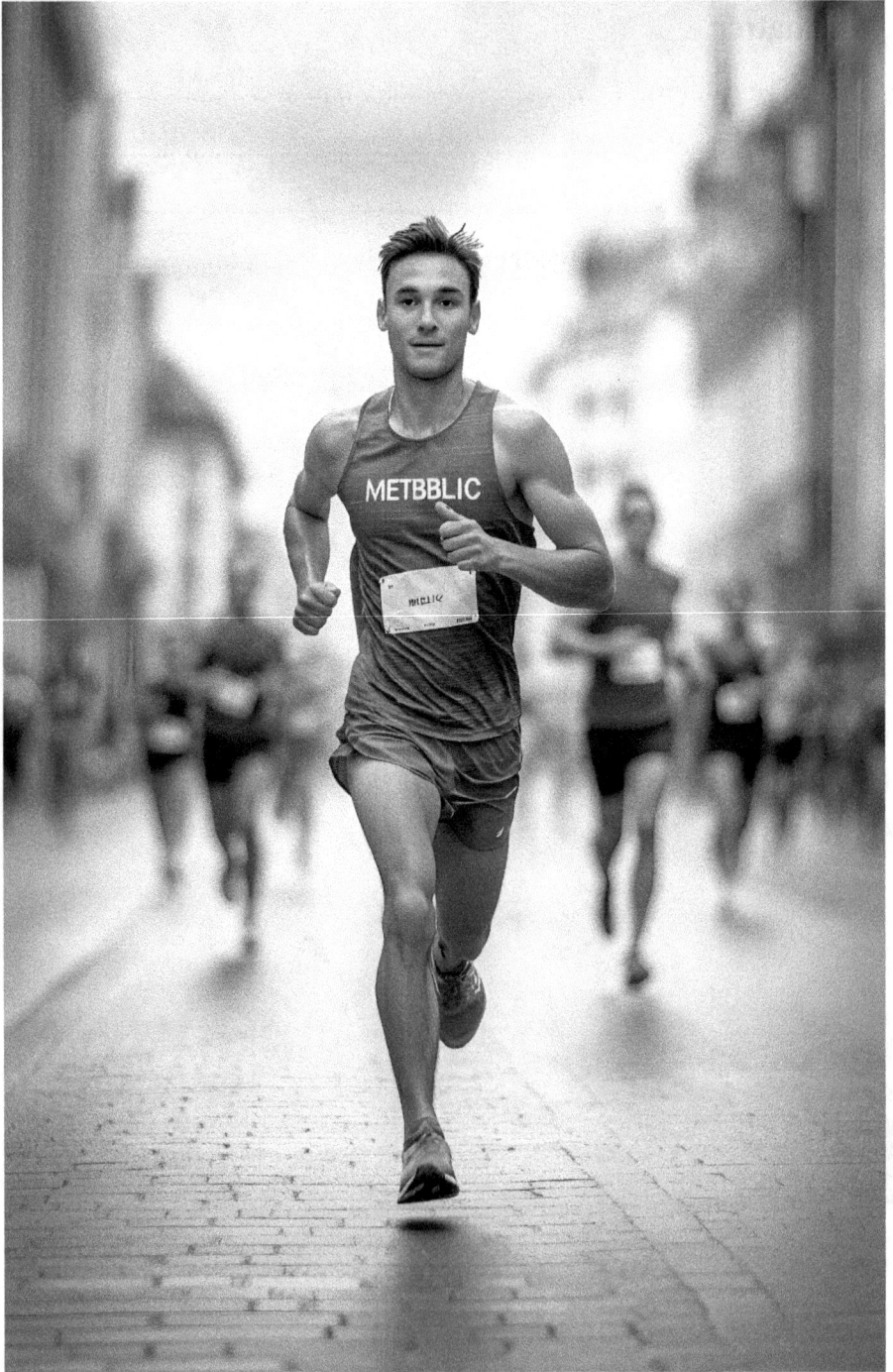

INTRODUCTION
&
BACKGROUND

About METBBLIC

At **METBBLIC**, we believe that health is personal, freedom is essential, and knowledge is power. Our approach—The METBBLIC Way—is a holistic, empowering philosophy designed to help individuals break free from industry-driven health myths and take full responsibility for their well-being.

At **METBBLIC**, our vision is to inspire and empower individuals to achieve *Better Being* (BB) by taking control of their health, optimizing their metabolism, and embracing personal responsibility. Our approach is rooted in four guiding pillars:

◆ MG – Metabolic Growth

We envision a world where individuals understand and harness the power of their metabolism to fuel energy, vitality, and longevity. By prioritizing metabolic health, people can break free from chronic fatigue, weight struggles, and industry-driven misinformation to reclaim their well-being.

◆ BT – Better Tomorrow

Our mission is to help people build a better future through informed health choices. True transformation happens when we take control of our nutrition, lifestyle, and mindset, leading to a stronger, healthier, and more vibrant life. METBBLIC is dedicated to equipping individuals with the knowledge and tools to create a sustainable path toward long-term wellness.

◆ BY – Build Yourself

Health is not something that happens to you—it's something you create. METBBLIC encourages self-improvement through conscious nutrition, strategic eating, and metabolic optimization. By taking ownership of one's health, every individual has the power to build a stronger body, a sharper mind, and a more resilient spirit.

◆ BB – Better Being

At the core of METBBLIC is the pursuit of a better and healthier way of living. Our vision is to make optimal health an achievable and enjoyable part of everyday life. We believe that by embracing metabolic truth, nutritional freedom, and personal responsibility, anyone can step into a life of strength, energy, and longevity.

These core aspects of the Vision of METBBLIC are reflected in our name and in our logo.

> *METBBLIC isn't just about health—*
> *it's about **Better Being, Better Tomorrow, and***
> ***Building Yourself for Metabolic Growth.***

The METBBLIC Way: A Framework for Thriving

Rather than following one-size-fits-all health advice, **The METBBLIC Way** encourages a metabolically intelligent approach to living. We focus on education, experimentation, and sustainability, enabling individuals to fuel their bodies for strength, energy, and longevity.

Our guiding principles

- **Personal Responsibility** – Your health is in your hands. Taking ownership of your choices is the first step to true wellness.

- **Education & Awareness** – Understanding metabolic health helps you make informed, independent decisions.

- **An Experimental Mindset** – No single diet or routine works for everyone. We encourage testing, tracking, and adapting based on real results.

- **Holistic Health** – Metabolism is the foundation of well-being. We integrate nutrition, movement, mental clarity, and longevity science for a complete approach.

- **Joy & Sustainability** – Health should be freeing, not restrictive. The best results come when you enjoy the process and build habits for life.

The Power of Metabolic Freedom

We believe that optimal health is possible for everyone—but only when you step outside the mainstream narrative. The medical, pharmaceutical, and food industries profit from disease management, not prevention. **The METBBLIC Way** is about reclaiming your right to vibrant, thriving health by fueling your body with what it truly needs.

Stepping into responsibility for your health is the first step toward the life you desire and deserve. No one can do it for you—but you already have the power to transform your health.

Live as if your health depends on it—because it does.

About this Book

This book expresses my experiences and point-of-view

The content os this book is derived from my own journey as I zig-zag a path that enables me to embrace and define **The METBBLIC Way**.

This book was produced with the assistance of AI

For this book, I worked with OpenAI's ChatGTP, Mistral.ai and Google's Gemini.

- I engaged in conversations with the ChatGTP to explore topics and situations of my selection.
- Most of the text of the sections were generated by the ChatGTP based upon my guidance, prompting, and requests for refinement.
- I reviewed, edited, and reformatted all of the text.

The perspectives presented are authentically my own.

How best to engage the content

You can peruse this book in any order that strikes you, including opening randomly, for you will find each page contains easily digestible and efficiently assimilable ideas and advice.

Disclaimer and a call for caution

I believe that a carnivore diet is better *for me*. It <u>may</u> offer potential benefits *for you*. My experience confirms the potential for reducing inflammation, improving metabolic health, and optimizing nutrient intake. However, as is often said, "your mileage may vary."

I am **not** a health practitioners and do **not** offer this book as medical advice. The following points <u>must not be understated</u>:

- The importance of developing a personal response relevant to your life situations.
- Giving mindful attention to potential illness considerations and/or nutrient deficiencies
- Developing a personal approach to adopting and maintaining a dietary practice, especially one as rigorous as Carnivore.

Consult with your Physician

- *It is important to consult with a healthcare professional before making any significant dietary changes, especially if you have pre-existing health conditions or are taking medications.*

- *The information presented here must not be considered medical advice.*

- *Consulting with qualified healthcare professionals is crucial for personalized guidance.*

Death is not an option, but Life (well lived) is

If you don't choose Life,

You'll get a laborious ride to death,

Which will come perhaps as a welcomed exit.

*To choose **The METBBLIC Way** is to choose Life.*

Why Nutrition and Health Myths Exist— And Who Benefits From Them

The world of nutrition and health is filled with myths, misinformation, and outright lies that have shaped public perception for decades. These myths are not random misunderstandings; they persist because they serve powerful interests that benefit from widespread confusion and dependency on their products and services.

1. The Food Industry: Profit Over Health

The processed food industry thrives on selling highly palatable, addictive, and nutrient-poor products. To sustain its profits, it promotes myths such as:

- *"Fat is bad for you"* – This myth allowed the rise of low-fat, high-sugar processed foods, which contribute to obesity and metabolic dysfunction.
- *"Whole grains are essential"* – A marketing ploy that justifies processed grain-based foods while ignoring their inflammatory and insulin-spiking effects.
- *"Plant-based is always healthier"* – A narrative that pushes highly processed meat substitutes while demonizing nutrient-dense animal foods.

Who benefits?

☞ Big Food corporations, agricultural giants, and manufacturers of ultra-processed, high-margin products.

2. The Pharmaceutical Industry: Disease Management, Not Health

The pharmaceutical industry profits from chronic illness—not from people being truly healthy. Myths that keep people sick and dependent include:

- *"High cholesterol causes heart disease"* – This myth fuels the multi-billion-dollar statin industry despite a lack of evidence that lowering cholesterol improves health.

- *"You need medication to control blood pressure, diabetes, and metabolic disorders"* – This belief keeps people reliant on drugs rather than addressing root causes through diet and lifestyle.

- *"Supplements and alternative health strategies are dangerous or ineffective"* – This discourages people from exploring holistic, nutrition-based solutions.

Who benefits?

☞ Pharmaceutical companies and the medical industry, which make money from lifelong medication use and chronic disease management.

3. Government & Public Health Policies: Controlled Narratives

Government health agencies often base their dietary guidelines on outdated, industry-influenced science, leading to myths such as:

- *"The USDA Food Pyramid is the ideal diet"* – A framework created with input from grain and processed food industries rather than unbiased nutritional science.

- *"Red meat and saturated fat are dangerous"* – Despite evidence that they provide essential nutrients, they are demonized due to flawed epidemiological studies.
- *"Calories in, calories out is all that matters"* – A simplistic and misleading approach that ignores the impact of hormonal and metabolic health.

Who benefits?

☞ Large-scale food producers, policy makers who serve industry interests, and organizations that depend on government funding.

4. The Media & Influencers: Clickbait and Corporate Influence

Sensational headlines and viral nutrition trends drive engagement and ad revenue, often at the expense of truth. Popular myths spread because:

- The media thrives on fear-based narratives (e.g., "Red meat causes cancer!").
- Sponsored content and influencer marketing promote misleading health trends.
- Social media algorithms favor controversy over accuracy, pushing myths that generate more clicks.

Who benefits?

☞ Media conglomerates, influencers paid by food and pharma industries, and online platforms profiting from engagement-driven misinformation.

5. The Fitness & Wellness Industry: Selling Trends, Not Solutions

Many fitness and wellness brands promote myths to sell diets, supplements, and programs, including:

"You need to eat every 2–3 hours to keep your metabolism high" – Encourages overconsumption and dependency on snacks and supplements.

"Detox teas, fat burners, and superfoods are necessary" – Fad-based products often lack real scientific support.

"All calories are equal" – Ignores the hormonal and metabolic impact of different macronutrients.

Who benefits?

☞ Supplement companies, fitness brands, and celebrity-backed wellness businesses profiting from misinformation.

Breaking Free from the Myths

To reclaim true health, individuals must take personal responsibility and seek unbiased, science-based truths rather than blindly trusting mainstream narratives. **The METBBLIC Way** is about breaking free from industry-driven deception, understanding what truly fuels the body, and making informed decisions based on metabolic truth, nutritional freedom, and strategic eating.

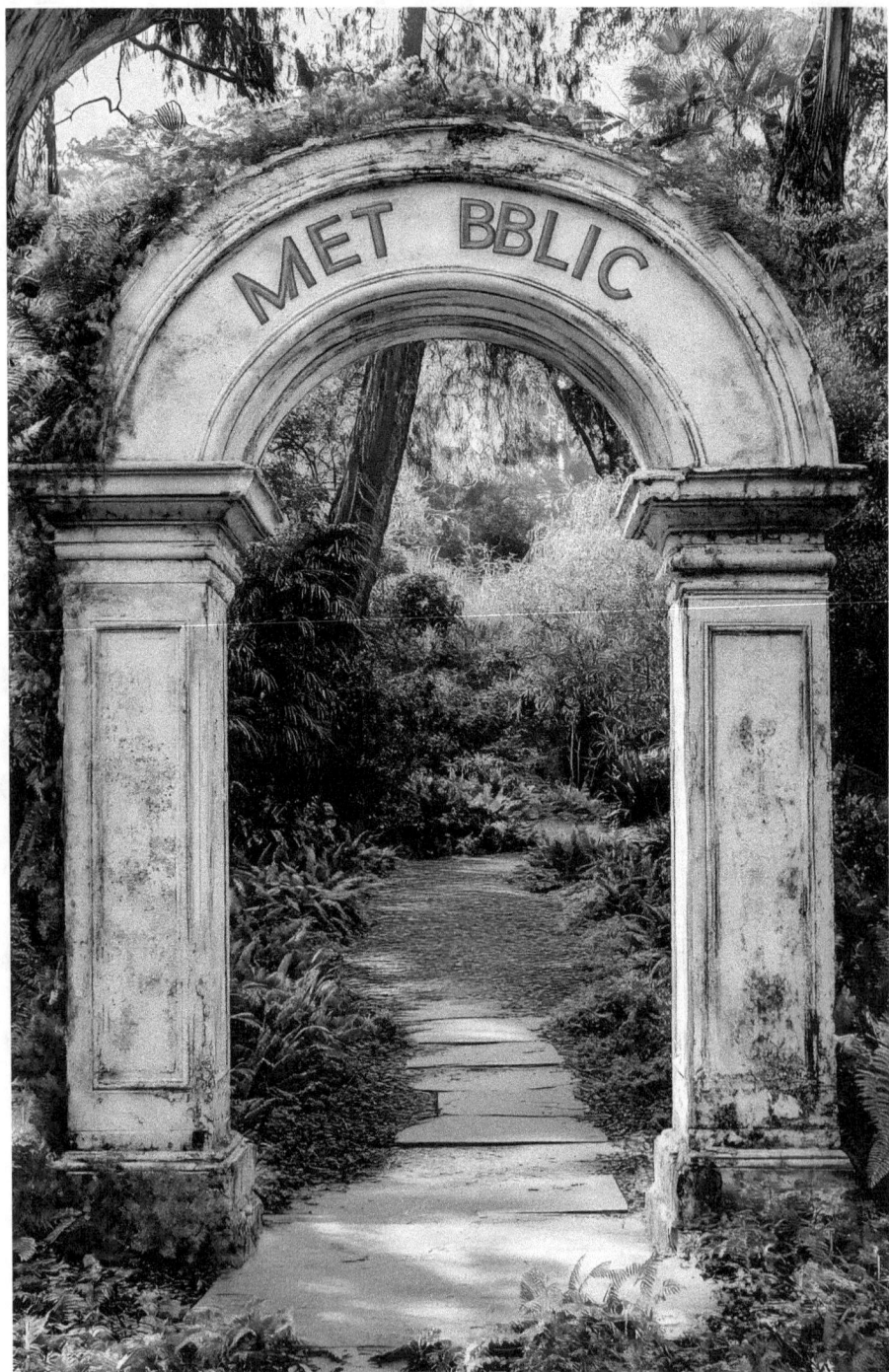

SECTION 1
CORE PRINCIPLES

THE FIVE CORE PRINCIPLES FOR METABOLIC WELLNESS AND VITALITY

1 Metabolic Truth

Understanding what truly fuels energy,
vitality, and longevity

🔍 Insight

Mainstream health advice has led people away from metabolic truth, promoting high-carb, low-fat diets that disrupt energy, hormone balance, and longevity. The body thrives on fat as its primary fuel, with protein as the foundation for strength and repair.

🧭 Orientation

Real health begins with metabolic efficiency—fueling your body with the right nutrients (animal-based proteins and fats) leads to sustained energy, mental clarity, and long-term vitality. Ditch the sugar-fueled rollercoaster and tap into your true energy source.

🌍 Context

For decades, mainstream health advice has promoted low-fat diets, calorie restriction, and plant-based eating as the path to longevity. Meanwhile, rates of obesity, metabolic disease, and chronic illness have skyrocketed. The reality? Much of what we've been told about nutrition and metabolism is misleading or outright false—crafted by industries that profit from sickness rather than health.

At METBBLIC, we focus on Metabolic Truth — the biological realities of how our bodies produce energy, build resilience, and sustain life. Metabolism is the foundation of strength, clarity, and longevity, and understanding it is the key to reclaiming your health.

📖 Summary

Metabolism is more than just burning calories — it's the process that powers every function in your body. When fueled correctly, your metabolism provides:

☑ *Sustained Energy* – No crashes, no dependence on stimulants.

☑ *Mental Clarity* – A sharp, focused mind free from brain fog.

☑ *Cellular Resilience* – Protection from aging, disease, and dysfunction.

☑ *Fat Adaptation* – Efficient use of stored energy, rather than constant hunger and cravings.

The truth? Humans thrive on nutrient-dense, bioavailable foods — not ultra-processed products or restrictive fads. The METBBLIC Way embraces animal-based nutrition, metabolic flexibility, and strategic fueling to optimize performance, longevity, and total well-being.

💡 Key Takeaway

When you understand your metabolism, you unlock true health freedom—free from industry myths, energy crashes, and chronic disease. Fuel your body the way it was designed, and you will thrive.

🚀 Call to Action: Embrace Metabolic Truth

- **Rethink Energy & Fuel:** Question conventional wisdom—fat, not carbs, is your body's most efficient energy source.
- **Track & Test:** Use tools like a CGM (Continuous Glucose Monitor) or ketone meter to understand how different foods impact your metabolism.
- **Ditch the Fear of Fat:** Saturated animal fats have been demonized unjustly—reintroduce them and observe the benefits.
- **Challenge the Calorie Myth:** Metabolism is not just about calories in, calories out—hormones, food quality, and metabolic flexibility matter more.
- **Heal Your Metabolism Naturally:** Reduce sugar, processed carbs, and inflammatory foods to restore metabolic health.
- **Prioritize Nutrient Density:** Choose foods rich in bioavailable vitamins and minerals—meat, eggs, and animal-based sources fuel vitality.
- **Take Ownership of Your Metabolic Health:** Doctors won't fix what poor diet and lifestyle created—only you can.

---

2 **Nutritional Freedom**

Breaking away from industry-driven
misinformation and restrictive dogma

🔍 Insight

The food and health industries profit from misinformation—keeping
people dependent on processed foods, pharmaceuticals, and dietary
myths. Nutritional freedom means breaking free from corporate-driven
dietary guidelines and reclaiming your right to eat for optimal health.

⏱ Orientation

Stop outsourcing your nutrition choices to industries that benefit from
your confusion. Nutritional freedom comes from questioning
conventional wisdom, experimenting with your diet, and embracing
what truly nourishes the body—without fear, guilt, or dogma.

🌐 Context

For decades, the food, pharmaceutical, and diet industries have dictated
what we "should" eat—promoting low-fat, high-carb diets, demonizing
animal fats, and pushing heavily processed "health" foods.
Governments, corporations, and mainstream media have reinforced
misinformation that keeps people trapped in cycles of poor health,
dependency, and chronic disease.

The result? Millions suffer from obesity, metabolic dysfunction, autoimmune disorders, and declining vitality—all while believing they're following the "right" diet. The truth is, much of modern dietary guidance isn't designed for health—it's designed for profit.

📖 Summary

Nutritional Freedom means breaking free from this system. It means:

✅ *Questioning the narrative* – Recognizing that mainstream advice is often biased and misleading.

✅ *Reclaiming ancestral wisdom* – Understanding that humans evolved thriving on whole, unprocessed, animal-based foods.

✅ *Ignoring restrictive fads* – Moving beyond calorie counting, guilt-based dieting, and unnecessary food fears.

✅ *Eating for optimal function* – Choosing nutrient-dense, bioavailable foods that fuel strength, clarity, and longevity.

True freedom comes from knowing what truly nourishes your body—without being manipulated by industry-driven trends, government food policies, or fear-based marketing.

💡 Key Takeaway

By freeing yourself from misinformation and restrictive dogma, you reclaim control over your health. You are not a customer for the disease industry—you are the architect of your own vitality.

🚀 Call to Action: Claim Your Nutritional Freedom

- **Break Free from Food Myths:** Challenge mainstream nutrition advice—trust results, not marketing or outdated guidelines.

- **Ditch Industry-Driven Foods:** Eliminate processed, artificial, and highly engineered products designed to keep you hooked.

- **Reclaim Your Intuition:** Learn to listen to your body's true hunger and satiety signals rather than following rigid dietary rules.

- **Define Your Own Optimal Diet:** Experiment with whole, unprocessed foods and track how they impact your energy, performance, and well-being.

- **Say No to Dogma:** Whether it's the plant-based push or calorie-counting obsession, free yourself from restrictive, one-size-fits-all nutrition advice.

- **Take Back Your Power:** Every bite you take is a choice—make it one that supports your vitality and longevity.

3 Personal Responsibility

Owning your health choices and outcomes

🔍 Insight

No one will care about your health more than you do. The system profits from disease management, not prevention—meaning you must take control of your diet, lifestyle, and mindset. Blaming genetics, circumstances, or bad advice keeps you trapped in poor health.

⏱ Orientation

Reclaiming your health starts with taking full ownership of your choices. When you prioritize knowledge, self-experimentation, and discipline, you break free from dependency on a failing system. No one is coming to save you—but you can save yourself.

🌐 Context

In today's world, many people unknowingly surrender control of their health to doctors, corporations, and government agencies. They follow standard medical advice, take prescriptions without question, and assume that their well-being is someone else's responsibility. But here's the truth: no one cares about your health as much as you do.

Modern healthcare is largely disease management, not true health optimization. If you rely on the system to "fix" you, you'll likely end up trapped in a cycle of medications, declining vitality, and frustration. The only way to break free is to own your health choices and outcomes — to shift from passive patient to active participant in your well-being.

📖 Summary

Personal Responsibility means recognizing that your health is in your hands. It's about:

✅ *Taking initiative* – Educating yourself instead of blindly trusting authority.

✅ *Making informed choices* – Understanding how food, movement, sleep, and stress affect your body.

✅ *Listening to your body* – Becoming attuned to what truly fuels you and what harms you.

✅ *Breaking free from victim mentality* – Refusing to blame genetics, aging, or bad luck for poor health.

While genetics and environment play a role, your daily choices determine your long-term health. Taking responsibility isn't a burden — it's the ultimate freedom.

💡 Key Takeaway

Your health is not the government's job, your doctor's responsibility, or an industry's priority. It's yours. The moment you accept this truth, you gain the power to transform your body, energy, and life.

🚀 Call to Action: Take Ownership of Your Health

- **Audit Your Health Decisions:** Assess your daily habits—are they moving you toward vitality or keeping you stuck?

- **Question the Narrative:** Don't accept conventional health advice at face value. Research, test, and trust your own experience.

- **Take Control of Your Inputs:** What you eat, read, watch, and believe shapes your health. Choose wisely.

- **Own Your Outcomes:** Instead of blaming genetics or circumstances, focus on what you can control—your actions and choices.

- **Make One Change Today:** Pick a single area (nutrition, movement, mindset, or sleep) and commit to improving it.

- **Stay the Course:** Health is a lifelong journey. Small, consistent efforts will create lasting transformation.

4 Strategic Eating

Learning how to nourish your body
for peak performance

🔍 Insight

Most people eat reactively—basing meals on cravings, habits, and misinformation. Strategic eating means fueling your body with intention—choosing foods that support energy, muscle function, cognitive clarity, and longevity, rather than just satisfying hunger.

⊘ Orientation

Food is either fuel or a burden. Eat with purpose—prioritizing nutrient-dense animal foods, healthy fats, and strategic timing to optimize metabolism, performance, and recovery. Your body is an engine—feed it what it was designed for.

🌍 Context

Most people eat reactively—driven by habit, cravings, emotions, or misleading nutritional advice. The food industry and mainstream health authorities push a one-size-fits-all approach that prioritizes convenience, processed options, and outdated dietary guidelines. As a result, people suffer from low energy, metabolic dysfunction, and chronic disease, never realizing that their food choices are keeping them trapped in poor health.

Strategic Eating flips this script. Instead of eating mindlessly or based on flawed recommendations, you fuel your body with intention and precision—choosing foods that maximize energy, metabolic function, and long-term vitality. Food isn't just about survival; it's a tool for performance, healing, and longevity.

📖 Summary

Strategic Eating is about making every bite count by:

✅ *Prioritizing nutrient density* – Focusing on whole, bioavailable foods that nourish rather than deplete.

✅ *Eliminating metabolic disruptors* – Removing inflammatory, toxic, and anti-nutrient-laden foods.

✅ *Aligning intake with energy demands* – Eating in a way that supports physical and mental performance.

✅ *Leveraging fasting and metabolic flexibility* – Understanding when and how to eat for optimal health.

This principle isn't about restrictive dieting—it's about precision and empowerment. When you fuel yourself strategically, you experience sustained energy, mental clarity, and resilience like never before.

Key Takeaway

Food is either fueling your strength or feeding disease. Strategic Eating is about taking control—choosing foods that work for your body, not against it, so you can operate at your peak every single day.

🚀 Call to Action: Master Strategic Eating

- **Prioritize Nutrient Density:** Focus on whole, bioavailable foods that fuel performance—primarily animal-based proteins and healthy fats.

- **Eliminate the Unnecessary:** Remove processed foods, excess carbohydrates, and inflammatory ingredients that drain your energy.

- **Eat for Function, Not Habit:** Tune in to true hunger signals instead of eating out of boredom, routine, or social pressure.

- **Experiment with Meal Timing:** Try fasting or adjusting meal frequency to optimize digestion, energy, and metabolic efficiency.

- **Listen to Your Body:** Track how different foods impact your energy, mood, and cognitive function—your body is the best feedback system.

- **Fuel with Purpose:** Every meal is an opportunity to build strength, resilience, and longevity—make your choices count.

5 Longevity & Performance

Thriving, not just surviving

🔍 Insight

Modern healthcare focuses on managing decline rather than maximizing vitality. True longevity isn't about just living longer—it's about maintaining strength, independence, and high performance at every stage of life.

🧭 Orientation

Longevity isn't about adding years—it's about adding life to those years. Prioritizing metabolic health, muscle preservation, and strategic lifestyle habits allows you to not just extend your lifespan, but enhance your healthspan. You're built to thrive—make choices that support that.

🌍 Context

Modern health advice is centered around disease management rather than true longevity and high performance. People are taught to accept fatigue, decline, and dependency on medication as inevitable parts of aging. But what if the goal wasn't just to avoid illness—but to optimize life?

Longevity isn't just about living longer; it's about living better. Performance isn't just about pushing harder; it's about functioning at your peak—mentally, physically, and metabolically—for as long as possible. When you understand how to nourish and care for your body correctly, you unlock the ability to extend both lifespan (how long you live) and healthspan (how well you live).

📖 Summary

The Longevity & Performance principle shifts the focus from mere survival to thriving by:

✅ *Optimizing metabolic health* – A well-functioning metabolism is the key to sustained energy, resilience, and a long, vibrant life.

✅ *Building strength and endurance* – Prioritizing muscle, movement, and metabolic efficiency to maintain peak performance as you age.

✅ *Eliminating metabolic slow poisons* – Avoiding the foods, habits, and toxins that accelerate aging and disease.

✅ *Harnessing regenerative practices* – Using fasting, sleep optimization, stress management, and strategic supplementation to extend healthspan.

Instead of coasting through life at half-capacity, this principle is about unlocking your full potential—living with vitality, strength, and clarity at every stage of life.

Key Takeaway

Longevity isn't just about adding years to your life—it's about adding life to your years. When you prioritize metabolic health, strength, and intelligent nutrition, you don't just extend your timeline; you elevate your entire experience of living.

Call to Action: Target Longevity & Performance

- **Track Your Energy & Recovery:** Pay attention to how you feel after meals, workouts, and sleep. Small adjustments can make a big difference.

- **Adopt a Longevity Mindset:** Think long-term. What daily choices can you make today that will benefit your future self?

- **Experiment & Adapt:** Try a new practice—like cold exposure, fasting, or movement variations—to see what enhances your resilience.

- **Measure What Matters:** Test key markers of health (strength, metabolic flexibility, sleep quality) rather than just weight or BMI.

- **Commit to Thriving:** Challenge yourself to elevate one area of performance this week—whether it's nutrition, movement, or mental clarity.

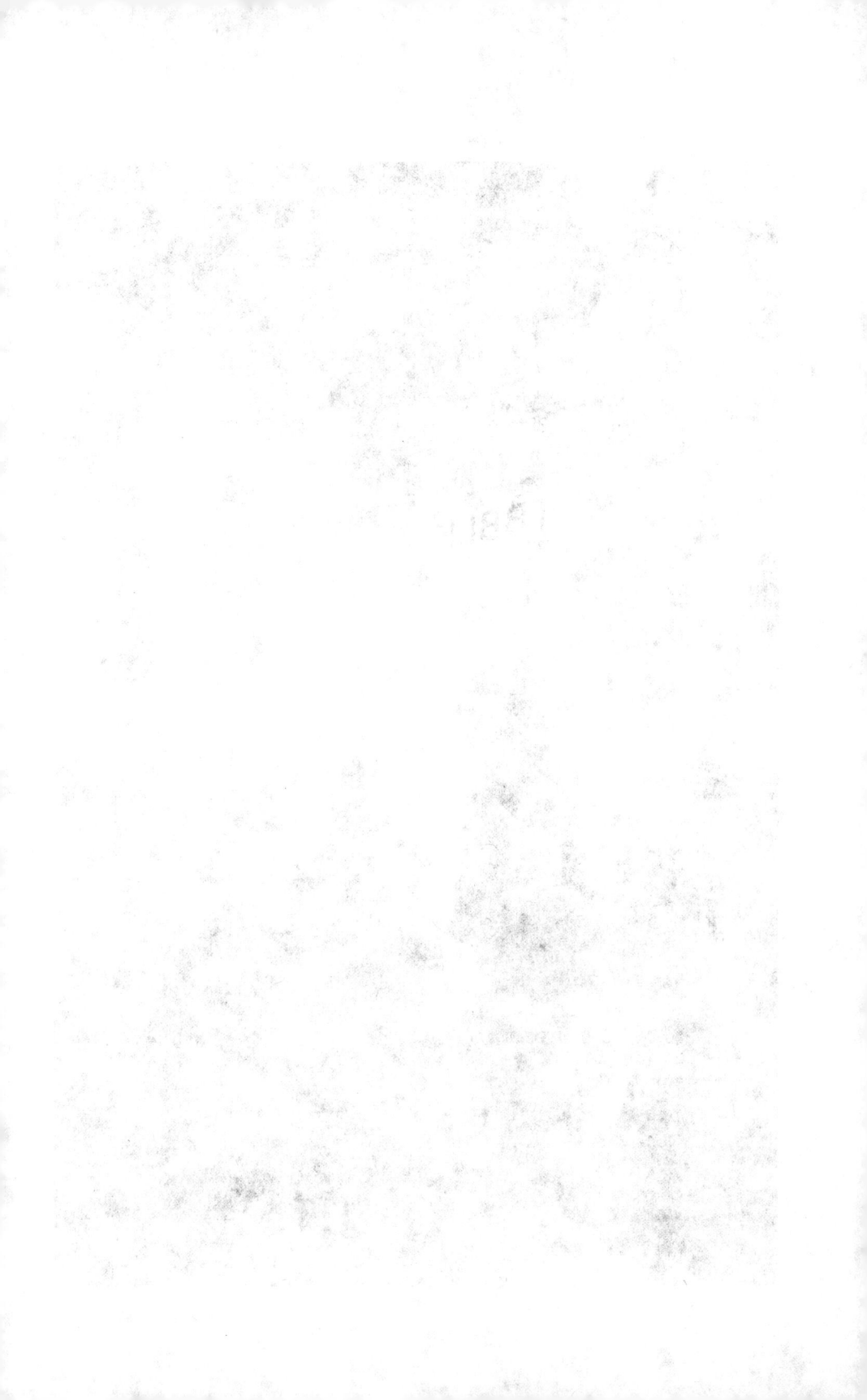

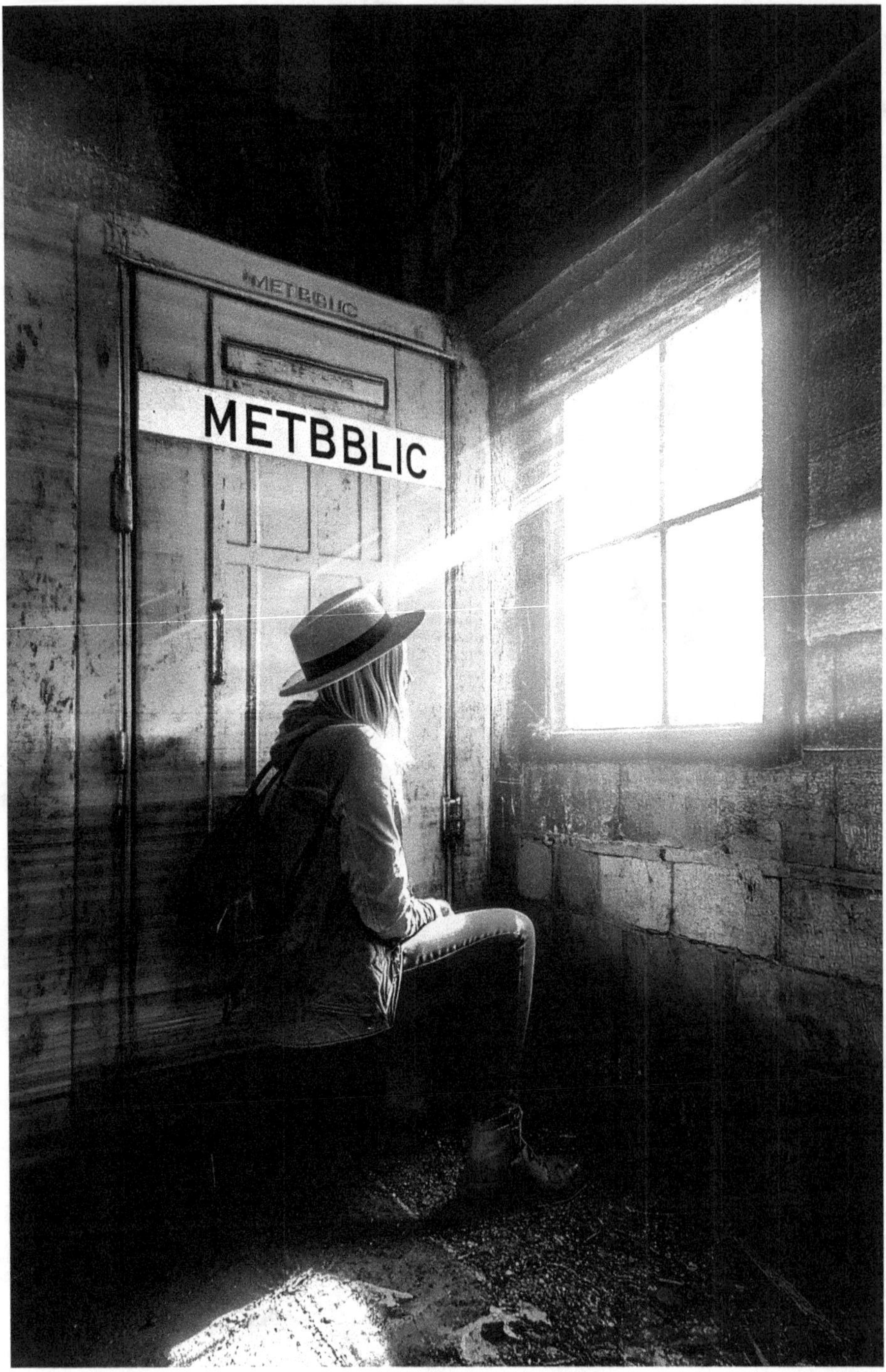
METBBLIC

SECTION 2
NUTRITIONAL FREEDOM

NUTRITIONAL FREEDOM REQUIRES BREAKING FREE FROM INDUSTRY-DRIVEN MYTHS

1 Cholesterol Causes Heart Disease

The war on cholesterol has led to misguided fear of animal fats, but the truth is LDL is not the enemy, and cholesterol is essential for hormone production, brain function, and cellular repair.

One of the most persistent and damaging myths in modern medicine is the belief that cholesterol causes heart disease. For decades, people have been told that eating cholesterol-rich foods and having high LDL ("bad" cholesterol) levels lead to clogged arteries, heart attacks, and strokes. However, this narrative is not supported by strong scientific evidence.

🔍 Where Did This Myth Come From?

The cholesterol-heart disease myth originated in the 1950s with researcher Ancel Keys, who promoted the idea that dietary fat, particularly saturated fat, raised blood cholesterol and led to heart disease. His infamous Seven Countries Study linked high-fat diets with heart disease, but he selectively chose data that fit his hypothesis while ignoring contradictory evidence.

Despite weak scientific backing, this flawed theory was adopted by governments, medical institutions, and the food industry. By the 1980s, low-fat diets were aggressively promoted, and cholesterol-lowering drugs (statins) became a multi-billion-dollar industry.

📍 The Truth: Cholesterol is Essential, Not Harmful

1. Cholesterol is NOT the Enemy

Cholesterol is a vital molecule necessary for:

✔ Cell membrane integrity – Every cell in your body needs cholesterol.

✔ Hormone production – Cholesterol is the building block for testosterone, estrogen, and cortisol.

✔ Vitamin D synthesis – Sunlight converts cholesterol in the skin into vitamin D.

✔ Brain function – Your brain is about 60% fat, with cholesterol playing a critical role in cognitive health.

2. No Proven Link Between Cholesterol & Heart Disease

- Large-scale studies have failed to show that high cholesterol directly causes heart disease.
- In older adults, higher cholesterol is associated with lower mortality.
- Many people who suffer heart attacks have normal or low cholesterol levels.

3. LDL is Not "Bad" – It Has a Purpose

LDL (low-density lipoprotein) is often demonized as "bad cholesterol," but in reality:

- LDL transports vital nutrients and energy to cells.
- It helps repair damaged tissues and inflammation in the body.

The real issue is oxidized LDL, which occurs due to sugar consumption, processed seed oils, and chronic inflammation—not dietary cholesterol.

4. The Real Cause of Heart Disease: Inflammation & Insulin Resistance

Instead of blaming cholesterol, the real culprits of heart disease include:

🔥 Chronic inflammation from processed foods, high sugar intake, and seed oils.

📈 Insulin resistance caused by excessive carbohydrates and metabolic dysfunction.

✏️ High triglycerides & low HDL (good cholesterol) – A much better predictor of heart disease than LDL alone.

💡 Who Benefits from the Cholesterol Myth?

💰 **Pharmaceutical Industry** – Cholesterol-lowering statins generate over $20 billion annually despite questionable benefits.

🍖 **Processed Food Industry** – Low-fat, high-carb products replaced traditional nutrient-dense foods, leading to an epidemic of obesity and diabetes.

🏥 **Medical System** – More "patients" means more lifelong medication and procedures rather than true health.

🔑 Key Takeaway: Cholesterol is NOT the Problem – Inflammation Is

- Cholesterol is essential for life – it does NOT cause heart disease.
- Low cholesterol is dangerous – linked to higher mortality, weakened immunity, depression, and cognitive decline.
- The real causes of heart disease are inflammation, insulin resistance, and metabolic dysfunction.
- LDL is not bad – but oxidized LDL (caused by sugar, seed oils, and processed foods) is harmful.

> *Instead of fearing cholesterol, focus on reducing inflammation, eating nutrient-dense foods, and optimizing metabolic health.*

2 Saturated Fat Is Bad for You

Decades of low-fat propaganda ignored the fact that saturated fat is a vital energy source, crucial for metabolic health, hormone balance, and brain function.

For decades, people have been told that saturated fat clogs arteries, raises cholesterol, and increases the risk of heart disease. This idea has driven dietary guidelines, food industry trends, and the widespread promotion of low-fat products. But the truth is very different. The fear of saturated fat is based on flawed science, misinterpretation of data, and corporate interests, rather than solid evidence.

🔍 Where Did This Myth Come From?

The demonization of saturated fat traces back to the 1950s, when Ancel Keys, a researcher, conducted the Seven Countries Study. His theory? That saturated fat raises cholesterol, which in turn causes heart disease.

🔋 What he didn't tell the world:

- He cherry-picked data from selected countries while ignoring others that contradicted his hypothesis.
- His study was purely observational, meaning it showed correlation, not causation.
- Many countries with high saturated fat consumption had low rates of heart disease, but these facts were ignored.

Despite its flaws, Keys' research shaped global dietary guidelines. By the 1980s, low-fat diets were aggressively promoted, and saturated fat was blamed for obesity and heart disease.

🍄 The Truth: Saturated Fat is NOT Dangerous

1. No Proven Link Between Saturated Fat & Heart Disease

- Multiple large-scale studies have failed to prove that saturated fat causes heart disease.

- A 2010 meta-analysis of 21 studies (American Journal of Clinical Nutrition) concluded: "There is no significant evidence that saturated fat is associated with an increased risk of heart disease."

- The PURE study (2017), which included 135,000 participants, found higher saturated fat intake was associated with lower mortality risk.

2. Saturated Fat is Essential for Health

Saturated fat is a necessary nutrient that supports:

✔ Brain Function – The brain is nearly 60% fat, with saturated fat playing a crucial role in cell integrity.

✔ Hormone Production – Testosterone, estrogen, and other hormones depend on cholesterol and saturated fat.

✔ Cell Membrane Health – Saturated fats are structurally stable, preventing oxidative damage.

✔ Strong Immune Function – Lauric acid (found in coconut oil) supports the immune system.

3. The Real Problem? Processed Carbs & Seed Oils

The rise in obesity, diabetes, and heart disease correlates not with saturated fat consumption, but with:

High-Carbohydrate Diets – Increased insulin resistance and inflammation.

Processed Seed Oils – Promote oxidative stress and arterial damage.

Sugar & Ultra-Processed Foods – Major drivers of metabolic disease.

4. The Food Industry's Role in the Saturated Fat Myth

When saturated fat was wrongly demonized, food companies replaced natural fats with hydrogenated oils, trans fats, and refined carbohydrates – leading to a surge in obesity, diabetes, and chronic disease.

Low-fat products = Higher sugar content = More metabolic disease.

Seed oil industry profits soared as cheap vegetable oils replaced butter and animal fats.

Statin drugs became a multi-billion-dollar industry as people were told they needed to lower cholesterol.

Who Benefits from the Saturated Fat Myth?

Pharmaceutical Industry – Statins & cholesterol-lowering drugs generate billions in revenue.

Processed Food Industry – Low-fat, high-carb products = increased sales, higher profits.

Medical System – More sick people = lifelong dependency on medication & treatments.

Key Takeaway: Saturated Fat is NOT the Enemy

There is NO scientific proof that saturated fat causes heart disease.

- Saturated fat is essential for brain function, hormones, and metabolic health.
- The real culprits behind heart disease and obesity are sugar, processed carbs, and seed oils.
- Low-fat diets have made people sicker, not healthier.

> ✅ *Instead of avoiding saturated fat, embrace it from natural, whole-food sources like grass-fed meat, butter, eggs, and coconut oil for optimal health.*

3 Carbs Are Essential for Energy

Carbs Are Essential for Energy – The belief that you need carbohydrates for energy is a myth. The body runs efficiently on fat as a primary fuel source, leading to better endurance, stable energy, and mental clarity.

One of the biggest misconceptions in nutrition is the idea that carbohydrates are the body's primary and essential source of energy. We've been told that without carbs, we won't have enough fuel to function properly, leading to fatigue, brain fog, and poor performance.

But the truth is that carbs are NOT essential for energy or survival. The human body is fully capable of thriving without dietary carbohydrates, using fat and ketones as primary fuels.

🔍 Where Did This Myth Come From?

The belief that carbs are essential stems from outdated nutrition science, government guidelines, and food industry propaganda.

1. Misinterpreted Science

- The Dietary Guidelines for Americans (1977) recommended that 45–65% of daily calories come from carbohydrates, based on the assumption that glucose is the body's main fuel.
- Early studies showed that the brain uses glucose, leading to the incorrect assumption that we must eat carbs to provide it.

- Ignored Fact: The body can make all the glucose it needs from protein and fat through a process called gluconeogenesis.

2. Carbs = Cheap, Profitable Food

- The shift toward a high-carb, low-fat diet made way for processed foods, grains, and sugars, which are cheap to produce and highly profitable.

- The food industry promoted carbs as essential while demonizing fat, leading to rising obesity, diabetes, and metabolic disease.

3. Athletes and Endurance Myths

- Many believe that athletes need carbs for performance, but fat-adapted athletes can run on ketones more efficiently.

- The carnivore and ketogenic communities have proven that humans can perform at elite levels without carb dependence.

🍽 The Truth: Carbs Are NOT Essential

1. The Body Prefers Fat for Energy

Humans evolved to run on fat as the primary fuel source, with carbohydrates only playing a minor role in energy metabolism.

✔ Fat stores provide sustained energy, while carbs lead to blood sugar spikes and crashes.

✔ Ketones (produced from fat) are a cleaner, more efficient energy source than glucose.

✔ Long-term fat adaptation eliminates the need for dietary carbohydrates.

2. The Brain Does NOT Need Dietary Carbs

The brain does require some glucose, but that does not mean you need to eat carbs.

✔ The liver produces glucose through gluconeogenesis when needed.

✔ The brain runs efficiently on ketones, which reduce oxidative stress and inflammation.

3. Carbs Are Not Necessary for Muscle Growth or Exercise

- Protein and fat provide all necessary building blocks for muscle repair and energy.
- The body stores glycogen in muscles and the liver, which can be replenished without direct carb intake.
- Many elite athletes thrive on low-carb and carnivore diets with enhanced endurance and recovery.

4. Excess Carbs Contribute to Metabolic Disease

- Carbs are not essential, but they can be harmful in excess.
- High-carb diets lead to insulin resistance, diabetes, obesity, and inflammation.
- Low-carb diets, like Carnivore and Keto, have been shown to reverse metabolic disorders and improve overall health.

Who Benefits from the Carbohydrate Myth?

Big Food Industry – Carbs are cheap to produce and addictive, keeping consumers hooked.

Pharmaceutical Companies – More carbs = more insulin resistance, diabetes, and drug dependency.

Government Nutrition Guidelines – Promote grain-heavy diets, benefiting agricultural industries.

Key Takeaway: Carbs Are Optional, Not Essential

The body does NOT require dietary carbohydrates.

- Fat and ketones provide cleaner, more stable energy.
- The brain functions better on ketones than glucose.
- Excess carbs lead to metabolic disease, insulin resistance, and inflammation.
- You can thrive without carbs by prioritizing fat and protein as your primary fuel sources.

Embrace a low-carb, high-fat approach for optimal health, energy, and longevity!

4 | Red Meat Is Unhealthy

> *Despite fearmongering, red meat is one of the most nutrient-dense foods, providing bioavailable protein, B vitamins, iron, zinc, and essential fatty acids. The real culprit in chronic disease is processed food, not meat.*

For decades, we've been told that red meat causes heart disease, cancer, and early death. Health authorities, mainstream media, and dietary guidelines have demonized red meat, labeling it as a "dangerous" food that should be avoided or consumed in "moderation."

But the truth is the opposite. Red meat is one of the most nutrient-dense and health-supporting foods on the planet. The claims against it are based on flawed research, industry-driven misinformation, and biased nutritional guidelines.

🔍 Where Did This Myth Come From?

The fear of red meat comes from faulty epidemiological studies, misleading headlines, and corporate interests that benefit from shifting people toward processed, plant-based alternatives.

1. Flawed Observational Studies

- Most studies linking red meat to disease are epidemiological, meaning they rely on food surveys rather than controlled experiments.

- These studies fail to prove cause and effect—they only show weak correlations.
- People who eat more red meat often have unhealthy lifestyles (smoke more, exercise less, eat processed junk food).

2. The Saturated Fat & Cholesterol Myth

- Red meat was demonized alongside saturated fat, falsely blamed for heart disease.
- No solid evidence has ever proven that eating red meat causes heart disease.
- Cholesterol is essential for health, and saturated fat does NOT clog arteries.

3. WHO's Processed Meat & Cancer Scare

- The World Health Organization (WHO) classified processed meats as carcinogenic in 2015, leading to public panic.
- This was based on weak data and lumped fresh red meat together with processed meats containing harmful additives.
- No controlled trials have proven that unprocessed red meat causes cancer.

4. Big Food & Plant-Based Industry Influence

- The push against red meat benefits the processed food, grain, and plant-based industries.
- Fake meat companies, like Beyond Meat and Impossible Foods, profit from demonizing red meat while promoting ultra-processed, chemical-laden alternatives.

- Governments and corporations push meat taxes and "sustainability" narratives to shift dietary habits.

🍴 The Truth: Red Meat is a Superfood

1. Red Meat Provides the Most Bioavailable Nutrients

Red meat contains essential nutrients in their most absorbable form, including:

✔ High-Quality Protein – Contains all essential amino acids for muscle, repair, and metabolism.

✔ Heme Iron – The most absorbable form of iron, preventing anemia.

✔ B Vitamins (B12, B6, Niacin, Riboflavin) – Crucial for energy, brain health, and DNA repair.

✔ Zinc & Selenium – Boost immune function, hormone production, and antioxidant defense.

✔ Creatine & Carnitine – Enhance muscle strength, brain function, and energy metabolism.

2. Red Meat Does NOT Cause Heart Disease

- Studies blaming red meat for heart disease ignore the role of sugar, seed oils, and processed foods.
- Countries with higher red meat consumption (e.g., France, Argentina) do not have higher heart disease rates.
- The real cause of heart disease is chronic inflammation, insulin resistance, and seed oils—not red meat.

3. Red Meat is NOT Linked to Cancer

- The claim that red meat causes cancer is based on weak epidemiological studies with confounding variables.
- No study has ever proven that fresh, unprocessed red meat causes cancer.
- The real cancer risks come from processed foods, sugar, and toxins — not steak.

4. Grass-Fed vs. Grain-Fed: What Matters?

- Grass-fed beef has slightly more omega-3s and antioxidants, but ALL red meat is nutrient-dense.
- Even conventionally raised beef is far healthier than processed foods, grains, and fake meat.
- Eat the best quality you can afford, but don't fear red meat.

Who Benefits from the "Red Meat is Bad" Myth?

💰 **Big Food Industry** – Profits from selling cheap, processed, grain-based foods.

💰 **Plant-Based & Fake Meat Companies** – Push highly processed alternatives as "healthier."

💰 **Pharmaceutical Industry** – More metabolic disease = more drugs for diabetes, heart disease, and cancer.

💰 **Governments & Environmental Groups** – Promote "sustainable" diets that reduce meat consumption.

🔑 Key Takeaway: Red Meat is One of the Healthiest Foods You Can Eat

- Red meat is NOT unhealthy—it is a complete, nutrient-dense superfood.

- There is NO solid evidence that fresh red meat causes heart disease or cancer.

- The real dietary villains are processed foods, sugar, and seed oils.

- Demonizing meat benefits industries that profit from cheap, plant-based alternatives.

- A diet centered around red meat supports optimal health, strength, and longevity.

> ✅ *Eat red meat confidently—*
>
> *it's the food your body is designed for!*

5 Fiber Is Essential for Digestion

The idea that you must eat fiber to stay regular is misleading. Excess fiber can actually cause bloating, gas, and digestive issues, while a well-formulated diet can promote healthy digestion without it.

We've been told for decades that fiber is critical for digestion, gut health, and preventing disease. Health organizations and mainstream nutritionists insist that without fiber, you'd suffer from constipation, poor gut health, and even colon cancer.

But the truth is very different. While fiber can be beneficial for some people, it is not essential for digestion and can even be harmful for many. The idea that fiber is required for a healthy gut and regular bowel movements is based on flawed science, outdated assumptions, and industry influence.

🔍 Where Did This Myth Come From?

The fiber myth originated from weak epidemiological studies, the grain industry, and outdated beliefs about digestion.

1. The "Colon Cancer Prevention" Myth

- In the 1970s, British doctor Denis Burkitt claimed that Africans eating high-fiber diets had lower rates of colon cancer.

- His observational data was misinterpreted as proof that fiber prevents cancer.
- Modern controlled studies have found NO link between fiber intake and reduced colon cancer risk.

2. The "Fiber Cures Constipation" Myth

- Many people believe fiber is necessary for regular bowel movements.
- However, multiple clinical studies show that reducing or eliminating fiber often improves constipation.
- Fiber can actually cause bloating, gas, and digestive discomfort by fermenting in the gut.

3. Big Food and Grain Industry Profits

- The grain and cereal industries benefit massively from the fiber myth.
- Fiber-rich foods like whole grains, bran cereals, and plant-based products are marketed as "heart-healthy" despite causing digestive distress in many people.
- The promotion of fiber keeps processed food companies and pharmaceutical companies selling fiber supplements and laxatives.

  The Truth: Fiber is NOT Essential for Digestion

1. Fiber Can Worsen Constipation, Not Fix It

- Studies show that reducing fiber intake can dramatically improve constipation.
- A 2012 study found that patients who eliminated fiber had complete relief from bloating and constipation.

- Too much fiber bulks up stools excessively, leading to straining and discomfort.

2. No Scientific Evidence That Fiber Prevents Colon Cancer

- Large-scale studies, including a Harvard study on 88,000 women, found NO reduction in colon cancer risk from fiber.
- The real causes of colon cancer are chronic inflammation, processed food, and insulin resistance — not fiber deficiency.

3. Fiber Can Cause Digestive Issues

- Fermentable fibers (like those in beans and whole grains) can cause bloating, gas, and IBS symptoms.
- Insoluble fiber (from wheat bran) can be irritating to the gut lining.
- Many people feel better digestion, less bloating, and improved gut health when reducing fiber intake.

4. The Human Body is Designed to Function Without Fiber

- Carnivore and low-fiber diets have been shown to improve digestion, gut health, and bowel function.
- Inuit, Maasai, and other indigenous cultures thrive on animal-based diets with little to no fiber.
- Bowel movements continue normally even on fiber-free diets, proving that fiber is not essential.

💡 Who Benefits from the "Fiber is Essential" Myth?

💰 **Cereal & Grain Industry** – Profits from selling fiber-enriched "health foods."

💰 **Big Pharma** – Sells fiber supplements, laxatives, and IBS medications.

💰 **Plant-Based Food Companies** – Push fiber-heavy fake meat and plant-based foods.

💰 **Doctors & Health Organizations** – Promote outdated dietary guidelines based on weak science.

🔑 Key Takeaway: Fiber is NOT Essential for Digestion

- There is no scientific proof that fiber prevents constipation, colon cancer, or disease.
- For many people, reducing fiber improves digestion, bloating, and gut health.
- The need for fiber is an industry-driven myth, not a biological necessity.
- A well-formulated diet based on bioavailable nutrients (like animal-based foods) supports optimal digestion without fiber.

> ✅ *Don't fear a low-fiber diet—*
> *your digestion will likely improve without it!*

6 Vegetables Are Always Healthy

> *While some plants have beneficial compounds, many contain antinutrients (like oxalates, lectins, and phytates) that can impair digestion, block nutrient absorption, and cause inflammation.*

For decades, we've been told that eating more vegetables is the key to health and longevity. Governments, nutritionists, and mainstream health organizations promote the idea that a diet rich in vegetables is essential for disease prevention, optimal nutrition, and overall well-being.

But the truth is more complex. While some vegetables contain beneficial nutrients, they also contain anti-nutrients, toxins, and compounds that can cause inflammation, digestive distress, and nutrient malabsorption in many people. The idea that vegetables are always healthy is an oversimplification that ignores individual tolerance, metabolic health, and bioavailability of nutrients.

🔍 Where Did This Myth Come From?

1. The "Eat Your Greens" Public Health Campaign

- Public health authorities started promoting fruits and vegetables as essential to combat chronic disease.
- These recommendations were based on weak epidemiological studies, not controlled clinical trials.

- The assumption: Since vitamins and minerals exist in vegetables, they must be universally good for everyone.

2. The Misinterpretation of Epidemiological Studies

- Many associational studies claim that people who eat more vegetables are healthier.

- However, these studies fail to account for lifestyle factors—people who eat more vegetables also tend to exercise more, smoke less, and avoid processed foods.

- Correlation is not causation. No study proves that vegetables alone are the cause of better health.

3. The Plant-Based Industry & Food Companies

- The rise of veganism, plant-based movements, and corporate interests has led to aggressive marketing of vegetables as "superfoods."

- Processed food companies use plant-based health claims to sell fake meats, vegetable oils, and high-carb products as "healthy" alternatives.

- The demonization of meat further strengthened the "plants = good, animal foods = bad" narrative.

🍽 The Truth: Vegetables Are Not Always Healthy

1. Vegetables Contain Anti-Nutrients That Can Harm Health

Plants have evolved defensive chemicals to protect themselves from being eaten. Many of these compounds can be harmful to human health, especially in high amounts.

🚫 **Oxalates** (found in spinach, kale, almonds) – Bind to calcium and cause kidney stones, joint pain, and mineral deficiencies.

🚫 **Lectins** (found in beans, tomatoes, wheat) – Disrupt digestion, increase gut permeability, and contribute to autoimmune disorders.

🚫 **Phytates** (found in grains, nuts, legumes) – Block absorption of essential minerals like zinc, magnesium, and iron.

🚫 **Goitrogens** (found in cruciferous vegetables like broccoli and cabbage) – Can suppress thyroid function and contribute to hypothyroidism.

🚫 **Solanine & Other Nightshade Toxins** (found in potatoes, tomatoes, eggplants) – Can trigger joint pain, inflammation, and autoimmune reactions.

2. Nutrient Bioavailability Matters More Than Just Presence

- Just because a vegetable contains a nutrient doesn't mean your body can absorb it well.
- Many plant-based nutrients are in less bioavailable forms compared to animal foods.
- Iron in spinach (non-heme) is poorly absorbed compared to iron in red meat (heme iron).
- Vitamin A in carrots (beta-carotene) must be converted to retinol, whereas liver provides it directly.
- Proteins in vegetables are incomplete and less digestible than animal proteins.

3. Many People Feel Better When Reducing or Eliminating Vegetables

- Individuals with autoimmune diseases, IBS, and gut sensitivities often experience less bloating, inflammation, and fatigue on low-vegetable or carnivore diets.

- Removing high-oxalate foods (like spinach, almonds, and sweet potatoes) can resolve chronic pain and kidney stone issues.

- Many people thrive on animal-based diets with minimal or no plant intake.

Who Benefits from the "Vegetables Are Always Healthy" Myth?

💰 **Big Agriculture & Organic Farming** – Profits from selling vegetables, grains, and plant-based products.

💰 **Processed Food Industry** – Uses the "plant-based" trend to sell fake meats, vegetable oils, and ultra-processed foods as "healthy."

💰 **Supplement & Pharma Companies** – Sell fiber supplements, antacids, and medications for gut issues caused by plant toxins.

💰 **Vegan & Plant-Based Movements** – Push a narrative that supports their ideology while ignoring bioavailability and anti-nutrients.

🔑 Key Takeaway: Vegetables Are NOT Always Healthy for Everyone

- Many vegetables contain anti-nutrients that can block absorption of key minerals and cause inflammation.
- Some people thrive without vegetables and experience better digestion, energy, and mental clarity.
- Bioavailability matters more than just the presence of nutrients—animal foods are superior in nutrient absorption.
- The belief that vegetables are always healthy is an oversimplified, industry-driven myth, not a universal truth.

> ✅ *Eat vegetables strategically, based on your body's tolerance—not because you've been told they are necessary!*

7 You Need to Eat Multiple Small Meals Per Day

Frequent eating spikes insulin and prevents fat burning. Fasting and strategic eating patterns support metabolic health, longevity, and hormonal balance.

For years, we've been told that eating small, frequent meals throughout the day is the best way to maintain energy, boost metabolism, and prevent hunger. This advice has been repeated by nutritionists, fitness trainers, and health organizations, convincing people that skipping meals or eating less frequently will lead to slower metabolism, muscle loss, and energy crashes.

But the truth is quite different. There is no scientific basis for the claim that eating multiple small meals per day is inherently better than eating fewer, larger meals. In fact, this pattern can contribute to insulin resistance, digestive issues, and constant hunger cycles.

Where Did This Myth Come From?

1. Misinterpretation of Metabolism Research

- Many believe that eating frequently "stokes" the metabolic fire, but this is based on a misunderstanding of how metabolism works.
- Total daily energy expenditure (TDEE) depends on total food intake, not meal frequency. Eating 2,000 calories in six meals or two meals results in the same metabolic outcome.

2. The Fitness Industry & Bodybuilding Culture

- The idea of eating every 2-3 hours originated in bodybuilding communities that prioritize muscle gain and high-calorie intake.

- While this may work for elite athletes with extreme training regimens, it is unnecessary (and even counterproductive) for most people.

3. The Processed Food Industry & Snacking Culture

- The food industry profits from promoting frequent eating and snack consumption.

- Processed food companies push "healthy snacks" as essential for sustained energy—keeping people trapped in constant grazing habits that drive more sales.

🍴 The Truth: Fewer Meals Are Often Better for Health

1. Constant Eating Disrupts Insulin Regulation

- Every time you eat, insulin is released. Eating frequently keeps insulin levels elevated, preventing fat burning and increasing the risk of insulin resistance.

- Metabolic health improves with longer gaps between meals (e.g., intermittent fasting), which allows insulin to drop and the body to burn stored fat.

2. Meal Frequency Does NOT Boost Metabolism

- The idea that small meals increase metabolism is false.

- The Thermic Effect of Food (TEF) (the energy used for digestion) depends on total calorie intake, not meal frequency.

- Eating three 600-calorie meals has the same TEF as six 300-calorie meals.

3. Frequent Eating Can Lead to More Hunger & Overeating

- Small meals often fail to fully satisfy hunger, leading to constant cravings and mindless snacking.
- Fewer, larger meals allow for better satiety and natural appetite regulation through hormones like leptin and ghrelin.

4. Digestion Works Better with Longer Gaps Between Meals

- Frequent eating stresses the digestive system and can lead to bloating, acid reflux, and IBS.
- The Migrating Motor Complex (MMC), which cleans the gut between meals, only activates when fasting. Constant eating prevents this process, contributing to gut issues.

5. Eating Less Frequently Supports Fat Loss & Longevity

- Intermittent fasting and time-restricted eating have been shown to improve fat burning, cellular repair (autophagy), and longevity.
- People who eat fewer, nutrient-dense meals often experience better energy levels, mental clarity, and metabolic flexibility.

Who Benefits from the "Frequent Eating" Myth?

The Processed Food & Snack Industry – Profits from constant snacking and meal replacements.

The Supplement Industry – Promotes protein bars, shakes, and "metabolism-boosting" supplements.

💰 **Mainstream Nutrition & Fitness Media** – Keeps people hooked on complicated eating schedules instead of simple, effective approaches like intermittent fasting or nutrient-dense eating.

🔑 **Key Takeaway: You Don't Need to Eat All Day**

- Frequent meals do NOT boost metabolism—total calorie intake matters more.
- Eating constantly keeps insulin elevated, blocking fat burning.
- Longer gaps between meals support digestion, hunger control, and metabolic flexibility.
- Intermittent fasting or eating 2-3 well-balanced meals per day is often more effective for energy, fat loss, and health.

> ✅ *Eat when you're truly hungry,*
>
> *not just because the clock tells you to!*

8 Salt Is Bad for You

The real problem isn't salt; it's refined, processed food. Natural salt is essential for electrolyte balance, hydration, and nerve function.

For decades, we've been told that salt is dangerous—that it raises blood pressure, causes heart disease, and leads to water retention. This belief has led to widespread fear of salt, with health authorities recommending low-sodium diets and food companies pushing "low-salt" or "salt-free" products as healthier alternatives.

But the reality is that salt is an essential nutrient, not a dietary villain. While excessive sodium intake from processed foods can contribute to health issues, a well-balanced intake of natural salt is vital for metabolic function, hydration, and overall health.

Where Did This Myth Come From?

1. The Sodium-Hypertension Theory

- The belief that salt raises blood pressure and causes hypertension dates back to flawed studies in the mid-20th century.
- Early research linked excess salt intake to high blood pressure in a small group of salt-sensitive individuals but failed to account for other dietary and lifestyle factors.
- Later studies have shown that for most people, salt has little to no effect on long-term blood pressure.

2. The Processed Food & Fast Food Problem

- Many studies that link salt to poor health are actually looking at people who consume highly processed foods (loaded with sodium, refined carbs, and unhealthy fats).
- The real culprit behind metabolic disease isn't salt itself—it's the refined, ultra-processed junk food that comes with it.

3. The "Low-Sodium" Industry & Big Pharma

- The push for low-sodium diets has led to an explosion of "low-salt" and "salt-free" products that are often high in sugar and artificial additives.
- The pharmaceutical industry profits from the widespread use of blood pressure medications, many of which are prescribed due to the mistaken belief that dietary salt is the primary cause of hypertension.

🥄 The Truth: Salt is Essential for Health

1. Salt is Vital for Hydration & Electrolyte Balance

- Sodium is an essential electrolyte that helps maintain fluid balance, nerve signaling, and muscle function.
- Too little salt can lead to fatigue, muscle cramps, dizziness, and even cognitive impairment.

2. Salt is NOT the Primary Cause of High Blood Pressure

- Only about 25% of people are salt-sensitive, meaning most individuals can consume reasonable amounts of salt without significant blood pressure effects.

- High blood pressure is more strongly linked to sugar, processed food, stress, and poor metabolic health than salt intake.

3. A Low-Salt Diet Can Be Harmful

- Restricting salt too much can lead to:
- Fatigue & Weakness – Sodium is required for energy production and muscle function.
- Higher Risk of Heart Disease – Studies show that low sodium levels are associated with increased mortality, heart failure, and metabolic dysfunction.
- Insulin Resistance & Weight Gain – Sodium helps regulate insulin sensitivity and metabolic function.

4. Natural Salt is Different from Processed Sodium

- Table salt (highly refined sodium chloride) is stripped of minerals and often contains anti-caking agents and additives.
- Natural salts like sea salt or Himalayan salt contain trace minerals that support overall health.

Who Benefits from the "Salt Is Bad" Myth?

Big Food Companies – Sell processed low-sodium products that replace salt with MSG, sugar, and artificial additives.

The Pharmaceutical Industry – Benefits from increased use of blood pressure medications, diuretics, and other drugs.

Mainstream Health Organizations – Continue pushing outdated dietary advice while ignoring new research on metabolic health.

🔑 Key Takeaway: Salt is a Necessary Nutrient, Not a Villain

- **Salt** is essential for hydration, brain function, and overall health.
- **Processed foods**—not natural salt—are the real problem behind hypertension and metabolic disease.
- **Low-sodium diets** can cause more harm than good, leading to fatigue, insulin resistance, and increased risk of disease.
- Choose **high-quality, mineral-rich salts** (sea salt, Himalayan salt) and listen to your body's natural cravings for salt.

✅ *Salt is not your enemy—processed food is!*

9 Sugar in 'Moderation' Is Fine

Even small amounts of sugar can drive insulin resistance, inflammation, and metabolic dysfunction. Sugar isn't just empty calories—it's toxic to long-term health

The idea that sugar is safe when consumed in moderation is a misleading myth that ignores the addictive nature and cumulative harm of sugar. Even small amounts contribute to metabolic dysfunction, insulin resistance, and chronic disease over time.

Health authorities and food industries often promote the notion that "a little sugar won't hurt" and that it can be part of a balanced diet. However, this perspective ignores the biological effects of sugar, its addictive properties, and how even moderate consumption can lead to long-term health issues.

The Reality is that the idea that sugar is harmless when consumed in moderation is deceptive and dangerous. Even "small amounts" contribute to metabolic dysfunction, insulin resistance, and inflammation over time. Sugar is addictive, biologically harmful, and unnecessary in any amount.

🔍 Where Did This Myth Come From?

The sugar industry has spent decades manipulating public perception to downplay the dangers of sugar. In the 1960s, sugar industry-funded research blamed fat for heart disease while hiding sugar's role. Modern dietary guidelines still push the false idea that sugar can be safely consumed in moderation, despite overwhelming evidence of its harmful effects.

The food industry reinforces this myth because sugar makes processed foods more palatable and addictive, driving repeat purchases.

🍶 The Truth: Sugar is not essential for energy, metabolism, or health.

❌ Even moderate intake leads to blood sugar spikes, insulin resistance, and fat storage.

❌ Sugar disrupts hunger hormones, leading to overeating.

❌ Fructose in sugar overloads the liver, contributing to fatty liver disease and metabolic disorders.

❌ The body has zero biological need for added sugar.

Even a little sugar can fuel cravings, encourage overconsumption, and contribute to chronic disease over time.

◆ *Sugar is highly addictive.* Studies show that sugar activates dopamine and opioid receptors in the brain, similar to addictive drugs. This means "moderation" is a flawed concept, as even small amounts can trigger cravings and overconsumption.

◆ *Metabolic damage starts at low levels.* Every time you consume sugar, blood glucose and insulin spike, leading to inflammation, fat storage, and oxidative stress. Over time, even moderate sugar intake contributes to insulin resistance, obesity, and type 2 diabetes.

◆ *Sugar alters hunger and energy regulation*. Fructose, a key component of sugar, does not trigger satiety hormones like protein and fat do. This leads to increased hunger, more frequent eating, and greater calorie intake.

◆ *There is no biological need for added sugar.* Unlike protein and fat, sugar provides zero essential nutrients—only empty, addictive calories.

Who Benefits from the "Sugar in 'Moderation' Is Fine" Myth?

The Food Industry – Sugar enhances taste, extends shelf life, and increases product sales. Promoting "moderation" keeps people consuming sugar without guilt, ensuring steady profits for food manufacturers while fueling the chronic disease industry.

The Pharmaceutical Industry – More sugar consumption leads to more diabetes, obesity, and heart disease, keeping people on medications.

Health 'Experts' & Media – Companies and influencers sponsored by food corporations promote moderation to maintain sales.

This myth ensures sugar remains a staple in the modern diet, fueling both the food and medical industries.

🔑 Key Takeaway: Sugar is not safe in any amount

Sugar is a toxin, an addictive substance, and a metabolic disruptor. The moderation myth is a marketing ploy designed to keep people consuming just enough to stay addicted while thinking they're making a "healthy" choice.

🔥 Eliminate or minimize added sugars completely—aim for zero rather than moderation.

🔥 Read labels carefully—sugar hides under names like fructose, glucose, and maltodextrin.

🔥 Prioritize nutrient-dense whole foods—meat, eggs, and animal fats provide all the energy you need.

🔥 Break free from sugar addiction—once removed, your cravings and energy fluctuations will disappear.

📌 Take Note

The belief that sugar is fine in moderation is misleading because:

- Sugar is addictive, making moderation difficult.
- Even small amounts contribute to metabolic disease over time.
- Sugar disrupts hormonal regulation, leading to overeating and fat gain.
- There is no safe threshold—each dose of sugar adds unnecessary stress to the body.

Rather than focusing on "moderation," the best approach is to minimize or eliminate added sugar entirely. "Moderation" is a marketing tactic, not a scientific truth. Sugar is harmful in any amount, and the best way to protect your health, metabolism, and longevity is to avoid it whenever possible.

> ✅ *The best amount of sugar for optimal health?*
>
> *ZERO.*

10 Calories In, Calories Out Is All That Matters

Metabolism is not just a math equation. Hormones, food quality, and nutrient timing matter more than just cutting calories. Not all calories are equal.

The mainstream weight-loss industry has long pushed the idea that all you need to do to lose weight is "eat less and move more." This belief is based on the principle of Calories In, Calories Out (CICO)—the idea that weight management is purely about the balance between calories consumed and calories burned.

But the reality is that human metabolism is far more complex than simple math. Not all calories are processed the same way in the body, and different foods trigger vastly different hormonal and metabolic responses.

🔍 Where Did This Myth Come From?

1. The Laws of Thermodynamics Misapplied

- The First Law of Thermodynamics states that energy cannot be created or destroyed—only transferred.
- While this law applies to closed systems like machines, the human body is not a closed system. It constantly adapts, adjusting metabolism, hormones, and energy expenditure based on food quality and composition.

2. The Diet Industry's Simplistic Approach

- CICO is an easy-to-sell concept—it sounds logical and straightforward, making it appealing to diet books, weight loss programs, and calorie-tracking apps.
- Many programs fail to address the role of hormones, nutrient quality, and metabolic adaptation, leading to repeated failure for dieters.

3. The Food Industry's Role

- The processed food industry promotes the idea that "a calorie is a calorie," allowing them to market highly processed, low-quality foods as "healthy" as long as they fit into a calorie-controlled diet.
- This ignores the hormonal and metabolic effects of different foods, which can drive hunger, fat storage, and disease.

🍴 The Truth: Food Quality & Hormones Matter More Than Just Calories

1. Different Macronutrients Affect the Body Differently

Macronutrient	Effect on Metabolism
Protein	Increases thermogenesis (burns more calories), supports muscle retention, and keeps you full.
Fat	Provides long-lasting energy, supports hormones, and does not trigger insulin spikes.
Carbohydrates	Easily stored as fat if not used immediately for energy, spikes insulin, and promotes hunger.

- 100 calories from steak ≠ 100 calories from soda.
- The body reacts very differently to processed carbs than it does to protein or fat.

2. Hormones Dictate Fat Storage & Weight Loss

- Insulin: High insulin levels promote fat storage and prevent fat burning. Processed carbs and sugars spike insulin, making it easier to gain weight.
- Leptin & Ghrelin: These hormones control hunger and satiety — processed foods disrupt these signals, leading to overeating.
- Cortisol: Chronic stress raises cortisol, leading to increased fat storage (especially around the belly).

3. Metabolism Adapts to Caloric Restriction

- Cutting calories drastically can slow metabolism, reduce energy levels, and increase hunger.
- The body responds by burning fewer calories, storing more fat, and increasing cravings.
- This is why most calorie-restricted diets fail long-term — they don't address the hormonal impact of food.

Who Benefits from the "Calories In, Calories Out" Myth?

The Processed Food Industry – Allows them to market ultra-processed, low-nutrient foods as "diet-friendly."

The Weight Loss Industry – Sells calorie-tracking apps, programs, and "low-calorie" processed foods.

💰 **Big Pharma** – Promotes weight-loss drugs and medications for obesity-related diseases caused by poor diet.

🔑 **Key Takeaway: Quality & Hormones Matter More Than Just Calories**

- *Not all calories are equal.* Food quality impacts hormones, satiety, and fat storage.
- *Weight loss is about metabolic health*, not just calorie math.
- *Highly processed carbs and sugars disrupt metabolism*, driving hunger and fat gain—even in a caloric deficit.
- *Focusing on nutrient-dense, whole foods* (especially protein and healthy fats) leads to sustainable weight loss and metabolic health.

> ✅ *Stop counting calories—start focusing on real, whole foods that support your metabolism!*

Why Nutrition and Health Myths Persist

Despite overwhelming evidence debunking many mainstream nutrition beliefs, myths about food, health, and metabolism continue to thrive. Why? Because the forces that shape public perception—big business, government policies, outdated science, and cultural norms—have a vested interest in keeping these myths alive.

Let's break down the key reasons why these myths persist:

1. Financial Interests: Profits Over Health

💰 The Processed Food Industry

- Multi-billion-dollar corporations profit from cheap, ultra-processed foods made with refined grains, sugars, and vegetable oils.
- They promote misleading health claims like "low-fat," "heart-healthy," or "fortified with fiber" to keep people buying their products, even when they contribute to disease.
- The myth that "a calorie is a calorie" allows them to sell processed junk as part of a "balanced diet."

💊 The Pharmaceutical Industry

- Chronic disease is profitable. The longer people suffer from obesity, diabetes, heart disease, and metabolic disorders, the more money is made from lifelong medications.

- Instead of promoting true health solutions like diet and lifestyle changes, pharmaceutical companies push drugs to manage symptoms — statins for cholesterol, insulin for diabetes, and blood pressure medications.

- They have no financial incentive to dismantle myths like "cholesterol is bad" or "saturated fat causes heart disease" because those myths justify their drugs.

🏛 Government & Health Organizations

- Government food policies are often shaped by corporate lobbying rather than science.

- The USDA food guidelines historically promoted grains and low-fat diets — not because they were healthy, but because of agricultural interests.

- Even after evidence disproves certain myths, policy changes are slow, as admitting past mistakes would damage credibility.

2. Outdated & Flawed Science

🔬 Early Misinterpretations of Data

- Many nutrition myths originated from flawed studies that were later debunked, but their influence remains.

- Example: The "cholesterol causes heart disease" myth came from the Seven Countries Study by Ancel Keys in the 1950s, which cherry-picked data to blame saturated fat for heart disease. Modern research has disproven it, but the myth still drives dietary guidelines.

Reductionist Science

- Nutritional science often studies food in isolation, ignoring the complex way foods interact in the body.
- Example: Studies on red meat fail to separate processed meats from fresh, grass-fed beef, leading to false claims that "meat is unhealthy."

Epidemiological Confusion

- Many "studies" that support nutrition myths are observational— meaning they show correlations, not causation.
- Example: If unhealthy people eat more red meat, it doesn't mean meat is the problem. People eating junk food and smoking may also eat meat, but the meat itself isn't causing disease.

3. Media & Misinformation

Sensationalized Headlines

- The media simplifies and exaggerates nutrition studies for attention-grabbing headlines.
- Example: "Eating eggs is as bad as smoking!"—a misleading conclusion from weak epidemiological data.

Social Media Virality

- Vegan and plant-based movements spread anti-meat propaganda that aligns with corporate interests (e.g., promoting fake meats like Beyond Meat).
- Influencers and celebrities often push trendy, misleading diets without scientific backing.

📚 Outdated Textbooks & Education

- Doctors and dietitians still learn outdated nutrition guidelines in medical school, reinforcing myths.
- Many nutrition programs are sponsored by food corporations that shape the curriculum.

4. Cultural & Psychological Conditioning

🥛 "We've Always Been Told This"

- If a belief has been repeated for decades (e.g., "milk is necessary for strong bones," "breakfast is the most important meal of the day"), it becomes deeply ingrained in society.
- Challenging these ideas makes people uncomfortable, even when new evidence proves them false.

🍩 Emotional Attachments to Food

- People don't just eat for nutrition—they eat for comfort, culture, and tradition.
- Myths like "vegetables are always healthy" persist because people associate them with virtue and morality.
- Admitting that a plant-based diet may be harming them is psychologically difficult for many.

🚫 Fear of Change

- Changing dietary beliefs requires breaking habits and confronting uncomfortable truths.

- Many people prefer to cling to familiar myths rather than overhaul their way of eating.

🚀 Breaking Free from Nutrition Myths

✅ *Question Everything:* Just because something is "common knowledge" doesn't mean it's true. Always ask, "Who benefits from this belief?"

✅ *Follow the Science, Not the Headlines:* Look at the quality of studies rather than relying on clickbait articles or cherry-picked data.

✅ *Eat for Metabolic Health, Not Industry Agendas:* Real, whole foods—meat, eggs, butter, and nutrient-dense animal fats—are the foundation of human health, no matter what the food industry says.

✅ *Be Your Own Experiment:* Instead of blindly trusting guidelines, test dietary changes yourself and observe how your body responds.

The Bottom Line

These myths persist because they serve powerful industries—not your health. Breaking free requires critical thinking, metabolic truth, and personal responsibility.

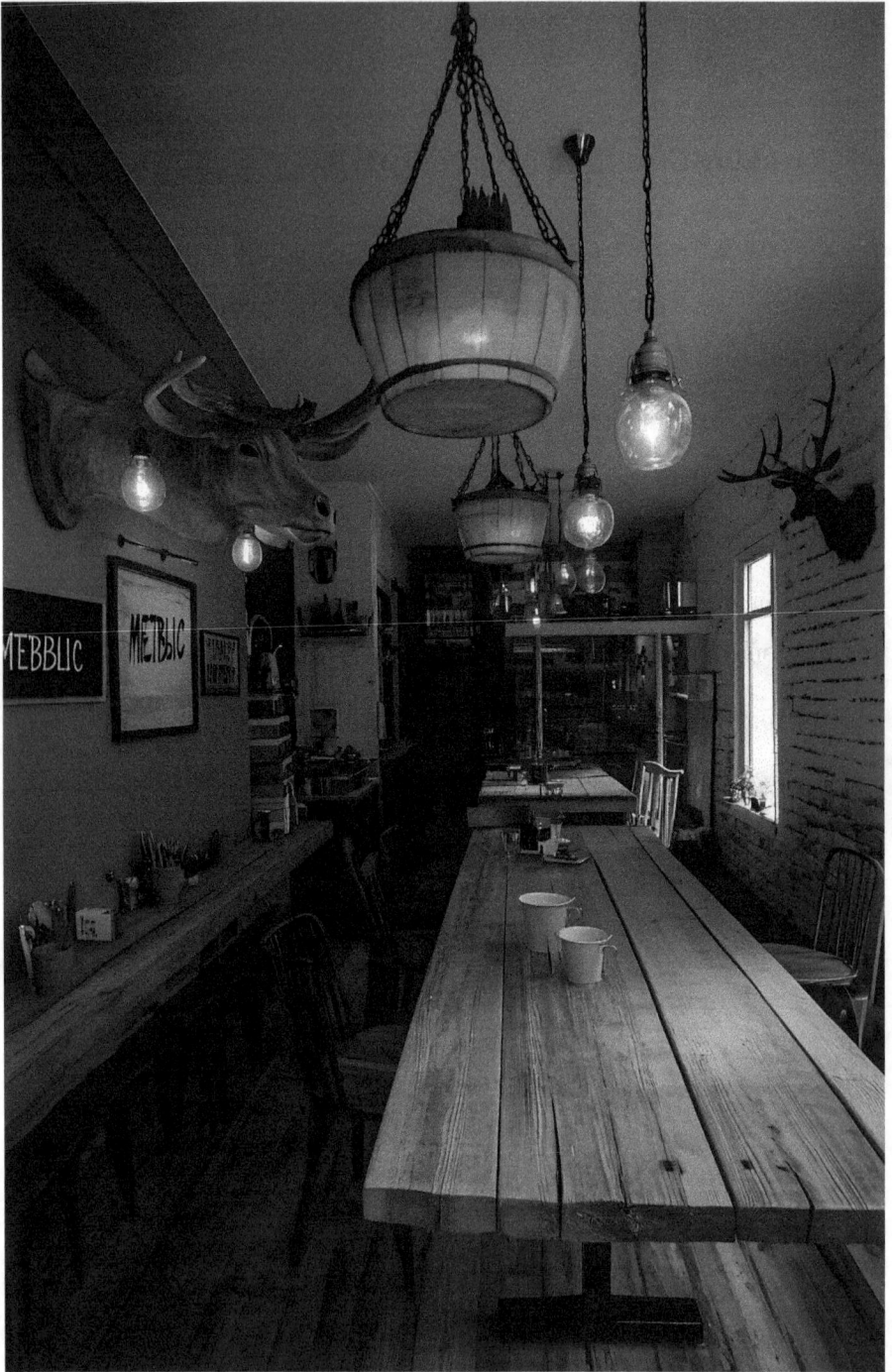

SECTION 3
FUEL YOUR BODY

HOW TO FUEL YOUR BODY FOR STRENGTH, ENERGY, AND LONGEVITY

1 Prioritize Animal-Based Nutrition

🔍 Why Animal-Based Nutrition?

Animal-based foods provide the most bioavailable and nutrient-dense sources of essential vitamins, minerals, and macronutrients. Unlike plant-based foods, which contain antinutrients that hinder absorption, animal foods offer complete proteins, healthy fats, and vital micronutrients in forms that the body can readily use.

🚀 The Power of Animal-Based Foods

Complete Proteins – Contain all essential amino acids in the right ratios for muscle growth, repair, and metabolic health.

Essential Fats – Provide crucial saturated and monounsaturated fats that fuel the brain, hormones, and cellular function.

Fat-Soluble Vitamins (A, D, E, K2) – These vitamins are found in egg yolks, liver, butter, and fatty meats, supporting immune function, bone health, and cardiovascular health.

Heme Iron & B12 – Found only in animal foods, these nutrients prevent anemia, boost energy, and support brain function.

Collagen & Glycine – Found in bone broth, skin, and connective tissue, essential for joint health, skin, and gut integrity.

🗑 The Pitfalls of Plant-Based Nutrition

Incomplete Proteins – Plant proteins lack essential amino acids and are harder to digest.

Antinutrients – Oxalates, lectins, and phytates block mineral absorption, leading to nutrient deficiencies.

Processed Fake Foods – Plant-based substitutes are often highly processed, full of additives, and low in bioavailable nutrients.

🍴 How to Prioritize Animal-Based Nutrition

◆ *Make meat the centerpiece of every meal*—beef, lamb, eggs, and fish are superior protein sources.

◆ *Incorporate organ meats* like liver for a nutrient boost.

◆ *Choose quality fats* such as butter, tallow, and ghee instead of vegetable oils.

◆ *Ditch plant-based fillers and ultra-processed alternatives* that lack real nutrition.

🔑 Key Takeaway

By fueling your body with animal-based foods, you give it exactly what it needs for energy, strength, and longevity—without the harmful effects of plant toxins and processed junk.

- *Meat, eggs, and animal fats* provide the most bioavailable nutrients for muscle growth, cognitive function, and metabolic health.
- *Red meat is a superfood*—rich in complete protein, B vitamins, iron, zinc, and essential fatty acids.
- *Avoid plant-based pitfalls*—antinutrients (oxalates, lectins, phytates) in many vegetables can impair digestion and nutrient absorption.

How Nutrient-Dense Animal-Based Foods Deliver Strength, Energy, and Longevity

Energy: Efficient and Sustained Fuel

Animal-based foods provide the most bioavailable and energy-dense sources of nutrition. Fats and proteins from animal sources are metabolized efficiently, providing long-lasting energy without the crashes associated with carbohydrates. Unlike plant-based foods, which often contain antinutrients that hinder absorption, animal products deliver readily usable fuel for the body.

- **Fat as the primary fuel:** Saturated and monounsaturated fats from animal sources offer stable energy, keeping blood sugar levels steady and avoiding insulin spikes.
- **Complete proteins:** Animal proteins contain all essential amino acids in the right ratios for energy production and muscle maintenance.
- **Ketogenic benefits:** High-fat, animal-based diets promote ketosis, a metabolic state where the body burns fat for fuel, enhancing endurance and mental clarity.

Strength: Muscle Growth, Repair, and Resilience

Strength comes from muscle and structural integrity, both of which require high-quality protein and essential micronutrients found abundantly in animal foods.

- **Protein for muscle synthesis:** Animal-based proteins contain high amounts of leucine, a key amino acid for muscle growth and recovery.

- **Collagen for joint and connective tissue health:** Bone broth, organ meats, and skin provide collagen, essential for joint strength, skin elasticity, and injury prevention.

- **Heme iron for oxygen transport:** Found only in animal products, heme iron is vital for red blood cell production, preventing fatigue and supporting endurance.

- **B Vitamins for strength and recovery:** B12, B6, and riboflavin in meat support cellular energy production and muscle repair.

⧖ Longevity: Cellular Health, Hormonal Balance, and Disease Prevention

- *Long-term health depends on reducing inflammation*, optimizing hormones, and protecting cells from oxidative stress—all of which animal-based nutrition supports.

- *Cholesterol for hormone production:* Found in animal fats, cholesterol is the building block of testosterone, estrogen, and cortisol, crucial for metabolism, muscle maintenance, and overall vitality.

- *Omega-3s for brain and heart health:* Fatty fish, egg yolks, and grass-fed meats contain EPA and DHA, essential for cognitive function, reducing inflammation, and cardiovascular protection.

- *Vitamin K2 for bone and arterial health:* Found in liver, egg yolks, and dairy, K2 directs calcium to bones rather than arteries, reducing the risk of osteoporosis and heart disease.

- *Retinol (Vitamin A) for immune function and longevity:* Preformed Vitamin A, abundant in liver and dairy, supports vision, immunity, and cellular repair—unlike beta-carotene from plants, which is poorly converted.

🔥 Bottom Line: Animal-Based Nutrition is the Key to Thriving

By prioritizing nutrient-dense animal-based foods, you provide your body with superior fuel for energy, complete proteins for strength, and vital nutrients for longevity. Unlike plant-based diets that rely on incomplete proteins and hard-to-absorb nutrients, animal-based nutrition supports optimal health at every level—from cellular repair to physical performance to long-term disease prevention.

> 👉 *Eat ancestrally, fuel optimally,*
>
> *and thrive effortlessly.*

2 Embrace Fat as Your Primary Fuel

🔍 Why Fat Over Carbs?

For decades, we've been told that carbohydrates are the body's primary energy source. This is a myth. The human body thrives on fat as its most efficient and sustainable fuel. Unlike carbs, which cause blood sugar spikes, insulin resistance, and energy crashes, fat provides stable, long-lasting energy while supporting metabolic health, brain function, and hormone balance.

🚀 The Benefits of Using Fat for Fuel

- **Sustained Energy** – Fat is slow-burning, preventing the energy crashes caused by carbs.
- **Metabolic Flexibility** – Teaches your body to use both dietary and stored fat for energy.
- **Improved Brain Function** – The brain runs efficiently on ketones, leading to better focus and mental clarity.
- **Hormonal Balance** – Cholesterol and saturated fats are essential for producing testosterone, estrogen, and cortisol.
- **Fat-Soluble Vitamin Absorption** – Vitamins A, D, E, and K require fat for absorption and utilization.

The Problem with Carbohydrates

- **Blood Sugar Rollercoaster** – Carbs cause energy spikes and crashes, leading to cravings and fatigue.
- **Insulin Resistance & Fat Storage** – Excessive carb consumption increases insulin levels, promoting fat storage and metabolic dysfunction.
- **Inflammation & Chronic Disease** – A high-carb diet contributes to obesity, diabetes, and cardiovascular disease.

How to Make Fat Your Primary Fuel

Prioritize Saturated and Monounsaturated Fats – Opt for butter, tallow, ghee, fatty cuts of meat, and eggs over vegetable oils.

Minimize Carbs – Reduce or eliminate sugar, grains, and processed carbohydrates to shift into fat-burning mode.

Increase Dietary Fat Intake – If you're feeling sluggish, eat more fat, not more carbs.

Use Intermittent Fasting – Fasting accelerates your body's ability to tap into fat for energy.

Key Takeaway

By embracing fat as your primary fuel, you reclaim your body's natural metabolic state, unlocking steady energy, mental clarity, and long-term health. Ditch the carb-dependency and fuel your body the way it was designed to function!

- Fat is the body's most efficient energy source, supporting stable blood sugar and sustained energy.
- Saturated and monounsaturated fats (found in beef, butter, tallow, and eggs) optimize hormone function, brain health, and cellular repair.
- Ditch industrial seed oils (canola, soybean, corn oil), which cause inflammation and metabolic dysfunction.

☞ *Be "Fat Adapted."*

You don't need sugar or carbs. Your liver can produce

all the glucose your body needs.

How Healthy Fats Deliver
Strength, Energy, and Longevity

⚡ Energy: Stable, Sustained, and Efficient Fuel

Healthy fats are the body's most efficient energy source, providing more than twice the energy per gram compared to carbohydrates (9 kcal/g vs. 4 kcal/g). Unlike carbs, which cause blood sugar spikes and crashes, fats offer a slow-burning, sustained energy supply, keeping you fueled throughout the day.

- **Ketones for optimal energy:** When fat is your primary fuel, your body produces ketones, a cleaner, more efficient energy source than glucose, reducing oxidative stress and brain fog.
- **No energy crashes:** Unlike carbohydrates, which lead to insulin spikes and energy dips, fats provide consistent energy without metabolic rollercoasters.
- **Mitochondrial efficiency:** Fats enhance mitochondrial function, helping your cells produce energy more efficiently and reducing metabolic damage.

💪 Strength: Muscle Maintenance, Recovery, and Resilience

Healthy fats are essential for muscle growth, repair, and hormonal balance, all of which contribute to physical strength and performance.

- **Testosterone and growth hormone production:** Saturated and monounsaturated fats support hormone synthesis, crucial for muscle growth, endurance, and recovery.

- **Cell membrane integrity:** Omega-3s and cholesterol strengthen cell membranes, improving muscle contraction, nerve signaling, and recovery.

- **Reduced inflammation:** Fats like omega-3s (EPA & DHA) from fatty fish and grass-fed meats reduce inflammation, protecting muscles and joints from injury.

- **Improved fat-soluble vitamin absorption:** Vitamins A, D, E, and K —critical for bone health, immunity, and recovery—are only absorbed in the presence of dietary fat.

⌛ Longevity: Cellular Protection, Brain Function, and Disease Prevention

Healthy fats play a critical role in protecting cells, reducing inflammation, and supporting longevity by keeping metabolic processes running smoothly.

- **Brain health and cognition:** The brain is nearly 60% fat, and consuming high-quality fats like DHA and cholesterol improves memory, focus, and protects against neurodegeneration.

- **Heart health and longevity:** Contrary to outdated dogma, saturated and monounsaturated fats increase HDL ('good' cholesterol) and improve lipid profiles, reducing cardiovascular risk.

- **Anti-inflammatory properties**: Fats from grass-fed meat, eggs, and wild-caught fish reduce systemic inflammation, the root cause of aging and chronic diseases.

- **Mitochondrial longevity:** Healthy fats reduce oxidative stress in mitochondria, preserving cellular function and delaying aging-related decline.

Bottom Line: Healthy Fats Are Essential for Thriving

Ditch the low-fat, high-carb lie—your body thrives on fat. By making healthy animal fats, omega-3s, and cholesterol the foundation of your diet, you unlock endless energy, enhanced strength, and true longevity.

> *Prioritize healthy fats, fuel your body right,*
> *and optimize your health for the long run.*

3 Control Carbohydrates Strategically

🔍 Why Carbohydrate Control Matters

Carbohydrates are not essential for human survival, but they can be used strategically based on individual goals, activity levels, and metabolic health. Uncontrolled carbohydrate consumption leads to insulin resistance, fat storage, inflammation, and chronic disease. Instead of mindlessly consuming carbs, strategic control allows you to optimize energy, performance, and longevity.

The Problem with Excess Carbs

- **Insulin Spikes & Energy Crashes** – Frequent carb consumption keeps insulin elevated, leading to blood sugar swings and fatigue.
- **Fat Storage & Metabolic Dysfunction** – Excess carbs get stored as fat, increasing the risk of obesity and type 2 diabetes.
- **Inflammation & Disease** – High-carb diets contribute to chronic inflammation, heart disease, and neurodegenerative disorders.

💡 How to Control Carbohydrates Strategically

◆ *Eliminate Processed & Refined Carbs* – Avoid sugar, grains, and ultra-processed foods that spike blood sugar and insulin.

◆ *Prioritize Low-Toxicity Carbs* – If consuming carbs, choose low-glycemic sources like berries or honey in moderation.

◆ *Time Carb Intake Based on Activity* – If you're highly active, consuming carbs post-workout may help with recovery.

◆ *Use Carbs as a Tool, Not a Staple* – Train your body to run on fat first and use carbs only when necessary.

Benefits from Controlled Carbohydrates

- **Fat Loss & Metabolic Health** – Low-carb approaches like Carnivore and Ketogenic diets improve insulin sensitivity.
- **Consistent Energy & Mental Clarity** – Reducing carb dependency prevents brain fog and mood swings.
- **Performance & Recovery** – Well-timed carbs can support athletic performance without disrupting fat adaptation.

Key Takeaway

Carbohydrates should be controlled, not mindlessly consumed. Prioritize fat for energy and use carbs strategically to avoid metabolic damage while optimizing performance and longevity.

- *Carbs are not essential*—the body can thrive on ketones from fat metabolism.
- *If consuming carbs, prioritize low-toxin sources* (e.g., raw honey, seasonal fruit) and time intake around activity.
- *Avoid sugar and processed grains,* which lead to insulin resistance, inflammation, and energy crashes.

How Controlling Carbohydrates Delivers Strength, Energy, and Longevity

Carbohydrates are often marketed as essential for energy, but uncontrolled carb intake leads to metabolic dysfunction, energy crashes, and chronic disease. By strategically managing carbohydrate consumption, you can optimize strength, maintain steady energy, and promote longevity.

💪 Strength: Muscle Preservation, Fat Adaptation, and Recovery

Carbs are not the body's primary fuel—fat and protein are. Proper carb control allows for metabolic flexibility, helping the body burn fat efficiently while preserving muscle.

- **Prevents Muscle Breakdown:** Excessive carbs cause insulin spikes, leading to fat storage rather than muscle building. Controlled intake allows for better hormonal balance, supporting lean muscle mass.
- **Optimizes Fat Adaptation for Strength:** When carbs are restricted, the body shifts to burning fat for fuel (ketosis), providing a consistent energy supply for endurance and performance.
- **Reduces Inflammation & Improves Recovery:** Processed carbs and excess sugar contribute to chronic inflammation, which slows down muscle recovery and weakens connective tissues.

Bottom line: Too many carbs impair strength by reducing metabolic efficiency and increasing fat storage instead of muscle development.

⚡ Energy: Stable Blood Sugar, Mental Clarity, and Consistent Performance

Carbs are often associated with energy, but the wrong kind and too many cause energy crashes, brain fog, and metabolic issues.

- **Prevents Energy Crashes & Sugar Spikes:** Processed and high-glycemic carbs cause rapid blood sugar spikes, leading to insulin overproduction, fatigue, and cravings.
- **Enhances Mitochondrial Efficiency:** By keeping carbs low, the body prioritizes fat oxidation, leading to more sustained energy production at the cellular level.
- **Improves Mental Focus & Cognitive Performance:** Excess carbs, especially sugar, impair brain function. Controlling carbs stabilizes brain energy levels, leading to better focus, memory, and cognitive endurance.

Bottom line: Controlling carbs results in consistent, long-lasting energy without crashes, improving both physical and mental performance.

⏳ Longevity: Metabolic Health, Disease Prevention, and Cellular Protection

Overconsumption of carbohydrates, especially refined ones, accelerates aging and increases disease risk. Strategic carbohydrate control supports metabolic health and cellular longevity.

Reduces Insulin Resistance & Prevents Diabetes: Chronically high carb intake leads to insulin resistance, increasing the risk of diabetes, obesity, and heart disease.

Minimizes Oxidative Stress & Inflammation: High carb diets, especially those rich in sugars, cause glycation (damage to proteins and DNA), accelerating aging and degenerative diseases.

Supports Longevity by Reducing Chronic Disease Risk: Controlled carb intake reduces the risk of obesity, cardiovascular disease, neurodegenerative disorders, and cancer.

Bottom line: Excess carbs fuel chronic disease and premature aging. Controlling them protects metabolic health, promotes cellular longevity, and extends lifespan.

🔥 Bottom Line: Carbohydrate Control is Key to Thriving

Build strength, sustain energy, and promote longevity by:

✅ *Prioritizing nutrient-dense, whole-food sources* (if consuming carbs at all!)

✅ *Eliminating refined sugars and processed carbs*

✅ *Using fat as the primary fuel source instead of glucose*

✅ A*dapting carbohydrate intake to activity levels* (low-carb for metabolic health, strategic carb use for performance)

☞ *Control carbs, stabilize energy,*

and unlock true vitality.

---

4 Focus on Protein for Strength and Vitality

🔍 Why Protein is Essential

Protein is the building block of life, essential for muscle growth, repair, and overall vitality. Unlike carbohydrates, protein is necessary for survival and supports metabolic function, immune health, and longevity. Prioritizing high-quality animal-based protein ensures optimal strength, satiety, and sustained energy.

The Problem with Inadequate Protein Intake

- **Muscle Loss & Weakness** – Inadequate protein leads to muscle wasting, weakness, and decreased resilience.
- **Slowed Metabolism** – Protein supports lean body mass, which keeps metabolism high. Low protein diets contribute to fat gain and metabolic decline.
- **Poor Recovery & Aging** – Insufficient protein impairs recovery, accelerates aging, and increases risk of osteoporosis and frailty.

📍 How to Optimize Protein Intake

🔶 *Prioritize Animal-Based Protein* – Choose beef, lamb, eggs, and seafood for complete amino acids and superior bioavailability.

🔶 *Eat Enough to Maintain Strength* – Aim for 0.8–1.2g of protein per pound of lean body mass to support muscle growth and repair.

◆ *Spread Protein Intake Throughout the Day* – Distribute protein consumption across meals to maximize muscle protein synthesis.

◆ *Avoid Incomplete & Low-Quality Protein Sources* – Plant-based proteins are inferior due to anti-nutrients, low bioavailability, and incomplete amino acid profiles.

Who Benefits from a Protein-Focused Diet?

- **Athletes & Active Individuals** – Protein supports muscle recovery, endurance, and performance.
- **People Focused on Fat Loss** – Protein increases satiety, preserves lean mass, and boosts metabolism.
- **Aging Populations** – Protein prevents sarcopenia (muscle loss with aging) and supports bone health.

Key Takeaway

Protein is essential for strength, longevity, and metabolic health. Prioritizing high-quality animal protein ensures muscle preservation, optimal recovery, and sustained vitality.

- *Protein is the foundation of muscle, longevity, and recovery.*
- *Aim for 1-1.5g of protein per pound of lean body mass* to preserve muscle and metabolic health.
- *Best sources:* Grass-fed beef, lamb, eggs, fatty fish, and organ meats.

> # How Strategic Protein Intake Delivers
> ## Strength, Energy, and Longevity

💪 Strength: Muscle Growth, Recovery, and Resilience

Protein is the foundation of muscle tissue, and consuming enough high-quality protein ensures optimal muscle growth, repair, and function.

- **Muscle Protein Synthesis (MPS):** Protein provides essential amino acids (EAAs), particularly leucine, which triggers MPS—the process that builds and repairs muscle.

- **Prevention of Muscle Loss (Sarcopenia):** As you age, muscle mass naturally declines. Adequate protein intake prevents muscle wasting, preserving strength and mobility.

- **Stronger Bones and Connective Tissue:** Collagen and amino acids like glycine support bone density, tendon strength, and joint integrity, reducing injury risk.

- **Enhanced Recovery & Reduced Soreness:** A well-balanced intake of animal-based proteins accelerates muscle repair, reducing inflammation and post-workout soreness.

⚡ Energy: Stable Fuel, Metabolic Efficiency, and Performance

While protein is not a primary energy source, it plays a vital role in metabolic function and energy production.

- **Blood Sugar Regulation:** Protein slows digestion, preventing blood sugar spikes and crashes that lead to fatigue.
- **Glucose via Gluconeogenesis:** In the absence of carbohydrates, protein can be converted into glucose only when necessary, ensuring steady energy without insulin surges.
- **Satiety & Appetite Control:** High-protein meals keep you fuller for longer, reducing cravings and helping with weight management.
- **Metabolic Boost:** Digesting and processing protein has a higher thermic effect (TEF) than fats or carbs, meaning it increases energy expenditure and promotes fat loss.

⧗ Longevity: Cellular Health, Hormonal Balance, and Disease Prevention

Protein is essential for repairing and maintaining every cell in your body, playing a critical role in longevity.

- **Hormonal Balance:** Protein supports the production of growth hormone, insulin, and neurotransmitters, all of which are essential for vitality and aging well.
- **Immune Function:** Amino acids are the building blocks of immune cells, helping your body fight infections and repair damage efficiently.
- **Collagen for Skin, Joints, and Organs:** Collagen and elastin maintain skin elasticity, joint function, and organ integrity, keeping you youthful.

- **Prevention of Chronic Disease:** Adequate protein intake reduces risk factors for metabolic syndrome, osteoporosis, and cognitive decline, all of which contribute to longevity.

Bottom Line: Strategic Protein Intake is Non-Negotiable

To build strength, sustain energy, and extend longevity, prioritize high-quality, animal-based protein sources such as beef, eggs, fish, and organ meats.

> *Eat protein with every meal, fuel muscle growth,*
>
> *and support a long, vibrant life.*

5 Optimize Electrolytes & Hydration

🔍 Why Electrolytes & Hydration Matter

Proper hydration isn't just about drinking water—it's about maintaining the right balance of electrolytes like sodium, potassium, and magnesium to support energy, brain function, and muscle performance. Without adequate electrolytes, dehydration can lead to fatigue, cramps, brain fog, and even serious health issues.

🔋 The Problem with Dehydration & Electrolyte Imbalance

- **Fatigue & Brain Fog** – Low electrolytes disrupt nerve signaling, leading to sluggishness and mental fatigue.
- **Muscle Cramps & Weakness** – Without enough sodium, potassium, and magnesium, muscles struggle to contract and relax properly.
- **Heart & Blood Pressure Issues** – Electrolytes regulate blood pressure and circulation. Imbalances can cause dizziness, irregular heartbeat, and low energy.
- **Mistaking Dehydration for Hunger** – Many people confuse thirst with hunger, leading to overeating and cravings.

💡 How to Optimize Electrolytes & Hydration

◆ *Prioritize Salt (Sodium)* – Natural salt supports nerve function, hydration, and blood pressure regulation. Don't fear salt—low sodium intake can lead to fatigue and dizziness.

◆ *Get Enough Potassium* – Found in meat, fish, and dairy, potassium helps regulate fluids, muscle contractions, and heart health.

◆ *Support with Magnesium* – Magnesium is essential for muscle function, relaxation, and stress management. Found in animal foods and supplementation if needed.

◆ *Drink to Thirst, Not Excessively* – Overhydration can dilute electrolytes, leading to imbalances. Sip water with electrolytes, especially when fasting or sweating.

◆ *Use Electrolyte Support When Needed* – If following a low-carb or carnivore diet, electrolyte needs increase due to lower insulin levels leading to faster sodium loss. Supplement with salt, potassium, and magnesium as necessary.

Who Benefits from Optimizing Electrolytes?

- **Anyone on a Low-Carb, Ketogenic, or Carnivore Diet** – These diets increase electrolyte loss, requiring higher sodium and potassium intake.
- **Athletes & Active Individuals** – Hydration and electrolytes enhance endurance, recovery, and muscle function.
- **People Experiencing Fatigue, Brain Fog, or Dizziness** – Often caused by electrolyte imbalances rather than actual dehydration.

🔑 Key Takeaway

Hydration isn't just about water—electrolytes are essential for energy, mental clarity, and muscle function. Prioritize sodium, potassium, and magnesium to maintain proper hydration and prevent fatigue, cramps, and sluggishness.

- *Salt is essential*—low sodium intake leads to fatigue, headaches, and poor performance.
- *Prioritize natural electrolytes* (sodium, potassium, magnesium) to support hydration, muscle function, and nerve signaling.
- *Drink water to thirst*, and include mineral-rich sources like bone broth.

☞ Read the ingredients!

Be careful of sugar, sweeteners and other additives that may be in commercial preparations.

How Proper Electrolyte Balance Delivers
Strength, Energy, and Longevity

Electrolytes—sodium, potassium, magnesium, and calcium—are the body's electrical signaling system. They regulate hydration, nerve function, muscle contraction, and cellular health, all of which are essential for strength, energy, and longevity.

💪 Strength: Muscle Function, Recovery, and Performance

Electrolytes are critical for muscle strength and function because they regulate nerve signaling and contraction.

- **Muscle Contraction & Prevention of Cramps:** Sodium, potassium, calcium, and magnesium ensure proper muscle contractions and prevent cramps, spasms, or weakness.

- **Faster Recovery & Reduced Soreness:** Magnesium and potassium help relax muscles post-exercise, reducing soreness and improving recovery time.

- **Strong Bones & Connective Tissue:** Calcium and magnesium play a role in bone mineralization and joint health, preventing fractures and stiffness.

Without balanced electrolytes, muscles become weak, coordination suffers, and performance declines—a direct hit to strength.

⚡ Energy: Cellular Hydration, Nerve Function, and Metabolic Support

Electrolytes regulate energy production at a cellular level, ensuring metabolic processes run efficiently.

- **Hydration & Nutrient Transport:** Sodium and potassium balance intracellular and extracellular water, preventing dehydration and fatigue.
- **Stable Energy & Mental Focus:** Electrolytes fuel the nervous system, allowing for sharp cognitive function, focus, and sustained energy.
- **Heart Function & Circulation:** Potassium and sodium regulate blood pressure and heart rate, ensuring oxygen and nutrients reach muscles and the brain efficiently.

Electrolyte imbalances lead to fatigue, dizziness, brain fog, and sluggish metabolism, draining your energy reserves.

⧖ Longevity: Cellular Health, Disease Prevention, and Anti-Aging

Long-term health depends on maintaining electrolyte homeostasis, which protects against disease and aging-related decline.

- **Prevention of Chronic Disease:** Low sodium levels have been linked to insulin resistance and metabolic syndrome. Magnesium deficiency is associated with higher risks of heart disease, osteoporosis, and neurodegeneration.

- **Cellular Integrity & Detoxification:** Potassium supports healthy kidney function, removing toxins and preventing fluid retention.

- **Reduced Inflammation & Oxidative Stress:** Magnesium helps regulate inflammation and supports mitochondrial function, the powerhouses of longevity.

Failing to replenish electrolytes can accelerate aging, cognitive decline, and metabolic dysfunction—all factors that shorten lifespan.

🔥 Bottom Line: Electrolytes Are Non-Negotiable

To build strength, sustain energy, and promote longevity, maintain proper electrolyte intake by:

✅ *Consuming enough sodium* (from natural salts)

✅ *Eating potassium-rich foods* (meat, seafood, dairy)

✅ *Ensuring magnesium intake* (meat, fish, organ meats)

✅ *Avoiding ultra-processed, high-sugar foods* that deplete electrolytes

---

> ☞ *Fuel your body with essential electrolytes*
>
> *and thrive.*

6 Implement Strategic Fasting

🔍 Why Fasting Matters

Fasting is more than just skipping meals—it's a powerful tool for metabolic health, fat loss, cellular repair, and longevity. Strategic fasting allows your body to shift from constant digestion to repair mode, improving insulin sensitivity, boosting energy, and enhancing mental clarity.

The Problem with Constant Eating

- **Blood Sugar Rollercoaster** – Frequent meals keep insulin elevated, leading to energy crashes, cravings, and fat storage.
- **Digestive Overload** – Your body spends too much time digesting and not enough time repairing.
- **Chronic Inflammation** – Constant feeding, especially with processed foods, contributes to inflammation and metabolic dysfunction.
- **Reduced Fat Burning** – Eating too often prevents the body from using stored fat for fuel.

♀ How to Implement Strategic Fasting

◆ *Start with 12–14 Hours* – A simple overnight fast (ex: 7 PM to 9 AM) allows the body to reset insulin levels and improve digestion.

◆ *Progress to 16–18 Hours* – Extending the fast increases fat burning (ketosis), mental clarity, and cellular repair (autophagy).

◆ *Use OMAD (One Meal a Day) Sparingly* – OMAD can be effective for weight loss but may not provide enough nutrients long-term.

◆ *Listen to Your Body* – Fasting is a tool, not a punishment. If you feel weak, adjust your approach (ensure adequate electrolytes and fat intake).

◆ *Break Your Fast Wisely* – Prioritize protein and healthy fats to avoid blood sugar spikes.

♀ Who Benefits from Strategic Fasting?

Anyone Looking to Improve Metabolic Health – Fasting reduces insulin resistance, inflammation, and oxidative stress.

People Struggling with Energy Crashes & Brain Fog – Time-restricted eating stabilizes blood sugar and enhances focus and mood.

Those Wanting Sustainable Fat Loss – Fasting allows the body to tap into stored fat for fuel without excessive calorie counting.

🔑 Key Takeaway

Fasting isn't about starvation—it's about timing your meals for maximum metabolic efficiency. Strategic fasting improves fat burning, mental clarity, and longevity while freeing you from the cycle of constant eating.

- *Intermittent fasting* (IF) and extended fasting enhance fat metabolism, cellular repair, and longevity.
- *Stop grazing*—eating constantly keeps insulin elevated and prevents fat burning.
- *Use fasting windows* (e.g., 16:8 or OMAD) to enhance energy, mental clarity, and metabolic flexibility.

How Strategic Fasting Delivers
Strength, Energy, and Longevity

Fasting is not starvation—it's a powerful tool that enhances metabolic efficiency, optimizes energy levels, and extends lifespan. You can maximize performance and well-being by implement strategic fasting.

💪 Strength: Enhancing Muscle Growth, Recovery, and Hormonal Balance

Contrary to the myth that fasting leads to muscle loss, strategic fasting actually supports muscle growth and recovery by optimizing hormones and cellular repair.

- **Boosts Growth Hormone for Muscle Preservation:** Fasting significantly increases human growth hormone (HGH), which helps build and maintain muscle while preventing muscle breakdown.

- **Enhances Fat Adaptation for Strength & Endurance:** With fewer insulin spikes, fasting trains the body to burn fat efficiently, providing a steady energy source for physical performance.

- **Increases Testosterone and Improves Recovery:** Fasting helps regulate testosterone levels, essential for muscle strength, endurance, and resilience.

- **Reduces Inflammation & Supports Faster Healing:** Fasting triggers autophagy, a process where the body removes damaged cells and regenerates new, stronger ones, improving muscle recovery and joint health.

Bottom line: Fasting preserves and strengthens muscle, optimizes fat burning, and enhances recovery.

⚡ Energy: Unlocking Sustained, Stable Power Without Crashes

Rather than relying on frequent meals for energy, fasting teaches the body to access stored fuel efficiently, resulting in stable and long-lasting energy.

- **Eliminates Energy Crashes & Sugar Dependence:** Without constant carb intake, blood sugar stabilizes, preventing insulin spikes and energy crashes.
- **Enhances Mitochondrial Function & Cellular Energy:** Fasting stimulates mitochondrial biogenesis, increasing the efficiency of energy production at the cellular level.
- **Boosts Mental Clarity & Focus:** During fasting, the brain shifts to using ketones, a more stable and powerful fuel than glucose, leading to enhanced cognitive function and mental performance.

Bottom line: Fasting provides stable energy, enhances brain function, and eliminates sugar-driven fatigue.

⧗ Longevity: Cellular Regeneration, Disease Prevention, and Lifespan Extension

Fasting is one of the most powerful longevity hacks, as it triggers deep cellular repair mechanisms that protect against aging and disease.

- **Activates Autophagy for Cellular Rejuvenation:** Fasting cleans up damaged cells, reducing the risk of cancer, neurodegenerative diseases, and premature aging.

- **Improves Insulin Sensitivity & Metabolic Health:** Strategic fasting lowers insulin levels, preventing diabetes, obesity, and heart disease.

- **Reduces Chronic Inflammation & Oxidative Stress:** Fasting lowers systemic inflammation, protecting against degenerative diseases like Alzheimer's, arthritis, and cardiovascular issues.

- **Enhances Longevity by Mimicking Caloric Restriction:** Studies show that fasting extends lifespan by improving metabolic function and delaying aging at the cellular level.

Bottom line: Fasting activates deep healing, slows aging, and protects against chronic disease.

🔥 Bottom Line: Fasting Unlocks Strength, Energy, and Longevity

By implementing strategic fasting, you can unlock the body's natural ability to heal, regenerate, and perform at its best.

✅ *Start with intermittent fasting* (12-16 hours fasting, 8-12 hours eating window)

✅ *Progress to longer fasts* (24-48 hours) for deeper autophagy and metabolic benefits

✅ *Break fasts* with nutrient-dense, animal-based meals

✅ *Listen to your body* and adapting fasting windows based on lifestyle and performance goals

> 👉 *Master fasting, unlock your true energy potential, and extend your healthspan.*

7 Eliminate Toxic & Processed Foods

🔍 Why It Matters

The modern diet is filled with chemically altered, ultra-processed, and artificial foods that wreak havoc on your health. Eliminating these toxic substances allows your body to function optimally, reducing inflammation, cravings, metabolic dysfunction, and chronic disease risk.

The Problem with Processed Foods

Loaded with Chemicals & Additives – Artificial flavors, preservatives, and seed oils contribute to inflammation, gut issues, and hormone imbalances.

Nutrient-Devoid & Calorie-Dense – These foods provide empty calories that spike blood sugar while lacking essential nutrients.

Engineered for Addiction – Processed foods are designed to trigger cravings and overconsumption, leading to poor metabolic health and weight gain.

Disrupts Gut Health – Industrialized ingredients damage the gut microbiome, contributing to digestive disorders, brain fog, and immune dysfunction.

Promotes Chronic Disease – Excessive consumption is linked to obesity, diabetes, heart disease, and neurological disorders.

What to Eliminate

◆ **Industrial Seed & Vegetable Oils** – Canola, soybean, sunflower, corn, and other seed oils cause oxidative stress and inflammation.

◆ **Refined Sugars & Artificial Sweeteners** – These spike insulin, damage metabolism, and promote insulin resistance, diabetes, and cravings.

◆ **Highly Processed Grains & Carbs** – White bread, pasta, and cereal are stripped of nutrients and cause blood sugar crashes.

◆ **Artificial Additives & Preservatives** – MSG, food dyes, and synthetic preservatives disrupt hormones and gut health.

◆ **Factory-Farmed, Low-Quality Meats** – Conventionally raised meats contain antibiotics, hormones, and inflammatory compounds.

Who Benefits from Eliminating Toxic & Processed Foods?

• **Anyone Seeking Long-Term Health** – Reducing processed foods lowers inflammation, stabilizes blood sugar, and supports metabolic function.

• **People Struggling with Cravings & Energy Crashes** – Whole foods provide sustained energy and reduce dependence on stimulants like sugar and caffeine.

• **Those Looking to Optimize Digestion & Mental Clarity** – Cutting out toxins heals the gut, reduces brain fog, and improves focus.

🔑 Key Takeaway

Your body is not designed to process fake food. Eliminating toxins, industrial oils, and processed junk allows your metabolism to function properly, reducing inflammation and promoting optimal energy, digestion, and long-term health.

- *Refined grains, seed oils, and processed sugars* are the primary drivers of chronic disease.
- *Avoid ultra-processed food products* marketed as "healthy" (plant-based meats, cereals, seed oils, protein bars).
- *Stick to whole, unprocessed animal foods* for maximum strength and vitality.

How Eliminating Toxic & Processed Foods Delivers Strength, Energy, and Longevity

The modern food industry is filled with ultra-processed, chemically altered, and nutrient-depleted products that are designed for profit, not health. Eliminating these toxic foods is one of the most powerful steps toward reclaiming your strength, sustaining high energy levels, and promoting longevity.

💪 Strength: Building a Resilient, Functional Body

Processed foods are loaded with inflammatory oils, artificial ingredients, and antinutrients that actively work against your body's ability to build muscle, recover, and perform at its best.

- **Removes Harmful Seed Oils That Cause Inflammation:** Industrial seed oils (soybean, canola, corn) contain high amounts of omega-6 fatty acids, which contribute to chronic inflammation, joint pain, and muscle soreness.
- **Supports Muscle Growth With Nutrient-Dense Whole Foods:** Processed foods lack bioavailable protein, essential vitamins, and minerals, leading to weaker muscles, poor recovery, and metabolic dysfunction.
- **Protects Against Gut Damage & Nutrient Malabsorption:** Additives, preservatives, and artificial sweeteners disrupt gut bacteria, impairing nutrient absorption and digestive function, leading to poor energy utilization and muscle fatigue.

Bottom line: Removing processed foods allows the body to absorb real nutrients, recover efficiently, and perform optimally.

⚡ Energy: Eliminating Energy Crashes & Optimizing Metabolic Function

Many processed foods are specifically engineered to be addictive while wreaking havoc on blood sugar, insulin levels, and metabolic function, leading to energy crashes and chronic fatigue.

Eliminates Blood Sugar Spikes & Crashes: Processed foods are typically high in refined sugars and fast-digesting carbs, causing rapid insulin spikes followed by extreme crashes, leading to fatigue and cravings.

Supports Mitochondrial Health for Efficient Energy Production: Artificial ingredients, preservatives, and chemical additives create oxidative stress, damaging mitochondria—the body's energy powerhouses.

Reduces Brain Fog & Enhances Mental Clarity: Processed foods often contain MSG, artificial dyes, and synthetic flavor enhancers, which impair neurotransmitter function, leading to brain fog, sluggishness, and poor focus.

Bottom line: Cutting toxic, processed foods stabilizes blood sugar, improves energy metabolism, and eliminates crashes and mental fatigue.

⏳ Longevity: Preventing Disease and Extending Lifespan

A lifetime of consuming processed foods leads to chronic diseases, metabolic disorders, and premature aging. Removing them enhances cellular repair, reduces inflammation, and supports long-term health.

- **Prevents Chronic Disease by Reducing Inflammation:** Seed oils, refined sugars, and artificial additives contribute to chronic inflammation, increasing the risk of heart disease, diabetes, and neurodegenerative conditions.
- **Lowers Cancer Risk by Eliminating Chemical Additives:** Many processed foods contain carcinogenic compounds like nitrites, acrylamide, and artificial preservatives, which increase cancer risk over time.
- **Slows Aging & Enhances Cellular Repair:** Processed foods accelerate oxidative stress and glycation, two major drivers of premature aging and cellular damage.
- **Supports Hormonal Balance & Metabolic Health:** Endocrine-disrupting chemicals in processed foods interfere with testosterone, estrogen, and insulin regulation, leading to hormonal imbalances and metabolic dysfunction.

Bottom line: Removing processed foods reduces disease risk, enhances longevity, and promotes optimal cellular function.

🔥 Bottom Line: Removing Processed Foods Restores Strength, Energy, and Longevity

To maximize your health, performance, and lifespan, eliminate:

❌ *Seed oils* (canola, soybean, corn, safflower, sunflower, peanut oil)

❌ *Refined sugar & artificial sweeteners* (high-fructose corn syrup, aspartame, sucralose)

❌ *Highly processed grains* (white flour, cereal, crackers, chips, industrial bread)

❌ *Artificial* additives, preservatives, and synthetic flavor enhancers

❌ *Factory-farmed*, chemically-laden meats and ultra-processed plant-based substitutes

---

👉 *fuel your body with whole, nutrient-dense,*
animal-based foods for strength,
sustained energy, and long-term health.

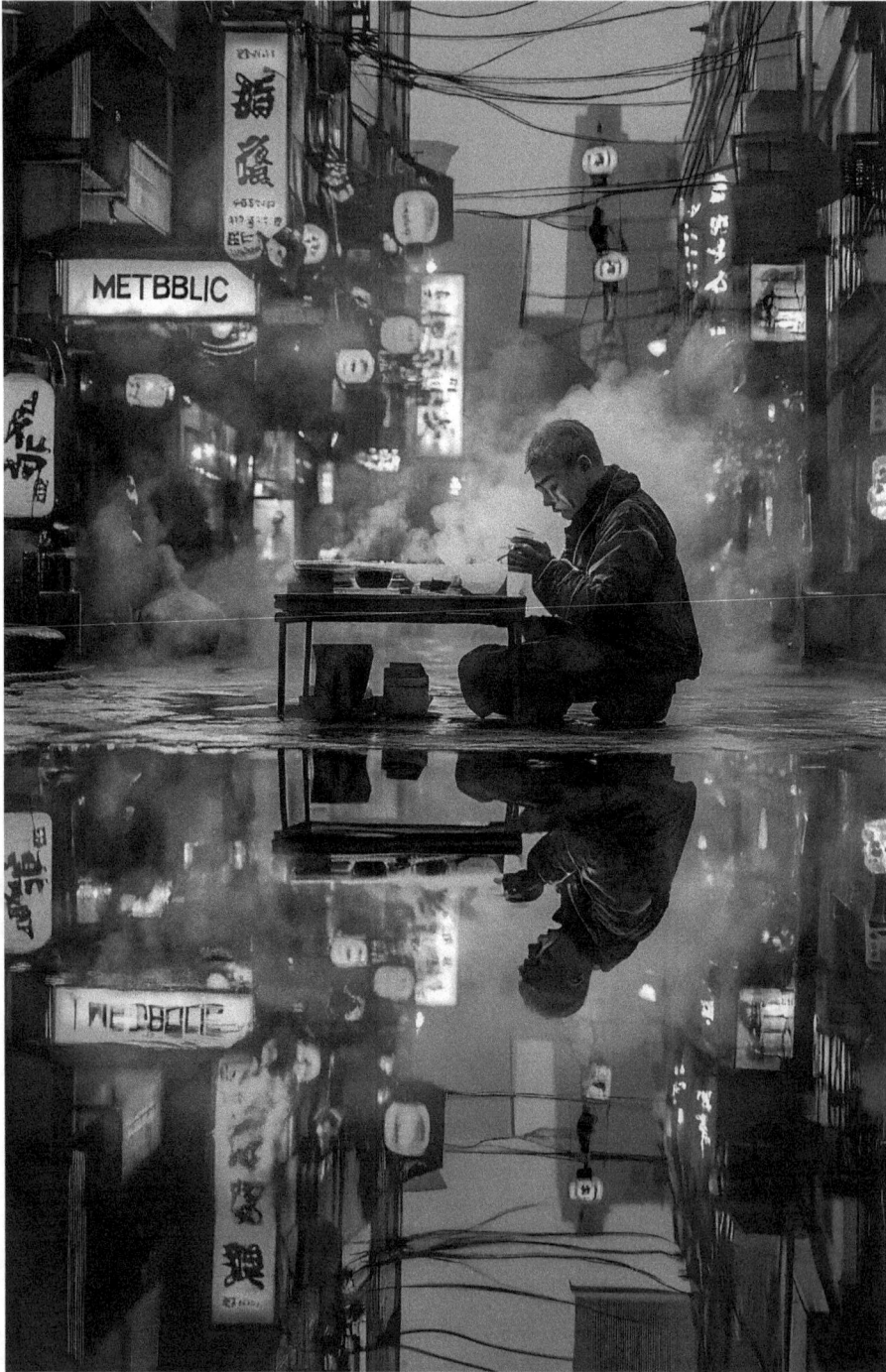

SECTION 4
PERSONAL RESPONSIBILITY

THE POWER OF PERSONAL RESPONSIBILITY IN RECLAIMING YOUR HEALTH

1 Own Your Health—No One Else Will

Personal responsibility is the foundation of true health and wellness.

In today's world, outsourcing your health to doctors, government guidelines, or food industry experts often leads to misinformation, chronic disease, and reliance on a broken system that profits from illness—not wellness. The harsh truth is: no one cares about your health as much as you do.

Taking ownership means questioning conventional wisdom, making informed choices, and committing to actions that serve your long-term well-being—because no one else will do it for you.

The Reality: The System Is Not Designed to Keep You Healthy

Most people blindly follow mainstream health advice, assuming it's in their best interest. However:

- *Doctors manage disease, not prevent it* – The medical system is reactionary, designed to treat symptoms rather than identify and eliminate root causes.
- *The food industry profits from addiction, not nutrition* – Ultra-processed foods are intentionally engineered to be addictive, leading to dependence on unhealthy diets.

- *Big Pharma thrives on lifelong customers, not cures* – Chronic illness is highly profitable, so there's little incentive to promote true health solutions.
- *Government health guidelines are influenced by industry interests* – Many dietary recommendations are shaped by food and pharmaceutical lobbies, not by unbiased science.

Relying on these institutions for health advice means handing over control of your well-being to entities that benefit from keeping you sick.

🍭 The Truth: You Are in Control of Your Health

Your health is not predetermined by genetics, age, or luck—it's the result of your daily choices, habits, and mindset. When you take full ownership, you:

- **Educate yourself** – Seek truth-based health knowledge rather than blindly following industry-driven narratives.
- **Take action** – Make intentional choices about what you eat, how you move, and how you live—because no one will do it for you.
- **Question authority** – If conventional health advice isn't working, challenge it, test new approaches, and find what actually works for your body.
- **Stop making excuses** – External factors don't dictate your health— you do. Instead of blaming circumstances, take proactive steps to improve your well-being.

Owning your health means shifting from dependence to self-reliance, victimhood to empowerment, and reaction to prevention.

Why This Matters for Strength, Energy & Longevity

When you own your health, you unlock:

Strength – A resilient, well-nourished body free from chronic pain, weakness, and disease.

Energy – Stable blood sugar, optimized metabolism, and a body that runs on real fuel, not stimulants or quick fixes.

Longevity – A lifestyle that prevents disease and supports long-term vitality, rather than just managing symptoms.

No one else will hand you optimal health—it's something you must claim for yourself.

Key Takeaway

Your health is your responsibility. No doctor, company, or institution will prioritize it for you. Educate yourself, take action, and make informed choices—because your life depends on it.

- The medical-pharmaceutical-food industry thrives on sickness, not health—profit is made by managing disease, not preventing it.
- Government guidelines and mainstream health advice are often driven by industry interests, not your well-being.
- Your health is your responsibility—no doctor, government agency, or corporation will care about it as much as you do.

✅ **Take Ownership Today**

Question conventional health advice—Does it serve your well-being, or does it serve industry profits?

Track your own health markers—Don't rely on standard ranges; understand what optimal levels look like for you.

Prioritize real food and lifestyle choices—Choose nutrient-dense, animal-based foods, movement, and metabolic health over convenience.

Commit to long-term health habits—Consistency, not quick fixes, leads to real results.

💡 *Bottom Line*

No one else will fight for your health—so you must. Take control, take action, and own your well-being.

2 Challenge the Health Dogma

Taking Personal Responsibility Means Questioning What You've Been Told

For decades, we've been fed health dogma that claims to be scientific, authoritative, and in our best interest—yet chronic disease, obesity, and metabolic dysfunction are at all-time highs. Clearly, something is broken.

Taking personal responsibility for your health means challenging the mainstream narrative, questioning who benefits from the advice you're given, and being willing to unlearn and relearn what actually leads to health, strength, and longevity.

The Reality: Most "Health Advice" Is Based on Profit, Not Science

Many health recommendations are not grounded in truth but in industry interests, outdated research, and misinformation that keeps people dependent on the medical-pharmaceutical-food complex. Consider these widely accepted myths:

Cholesterol causes heart disease – A narrative pushed by statin manufacturers despite no solid evidence linking dietary cholesterol to heart disease.

Saturated fat is bad for you – Demonized to promote low-fat, highly processed alternatives that make food companies billions.

Carbs are essential for energy – Encouraging people to rely on high-carb, insulin-spiking diets that drive metabolic disease.

Red meat is unhealthy – A claim based on weak epidemiology and corporate agendas, ignoring its nutrient-dense benefits.

Calories in, calories out is all that matters – A reductionist view that ignores metabolic and hormonal factors in fat storage and energy regulation.

This dogma is designed to keep you sick, dependent, and confused—so you continue consuming processed foods, medications, and unnecessary medical treatments.

📍 The Truth: Real Health Comes from Challenging the Narrative

You don't have to accept mainstream health advice at face value. Instead, take control by:

- **Looking at the real science** – Seek studies free from corporate influence, and evaluate research with skepticism.
- **Understanding conflicts of interest** – Follow the money. If an industry profits from keeping you sick, why would they promote true health solutions?
- **Testing things for yourself** – Your body is the best evidence. Try different approaches and assess how they actually make you feel.

- **Trusting ancestral wisdom** – Traditional diets based on animal-based nutrition, fasting, and whole foods have sustained human health for millennia—long before modern dietary guidelines.
- **Daring to think independently** – Don't let societal pressure or authority figures dictate your health choices. Question everything.

Taking responsibility requires courage—you must be willing to go against the grain, reject misleading mainstream advice, and stand by your personal findings.

Why This Matters for Strength, Energy & Longevity

When you challenge health dogma and seek truth-based nutrition and lifestyle habits, you unlock:

Strength – A body fueled by nutrient-dense, unprocessed foods, not weak from low-fat, high-carb misinformation.

Energy – Stable energy levels, free from the sugar crashes, inflammation, and metabolic dysfunction caused by conventional dietary recommendations.

Longevity – A lifestyle built on evolutionary principles that prevent disease rather than just managing symptoms.

Following mainstream health dogma leads to a lifetime of illness. Challenging it leads to true, vibrant health.

🔑 Key Takeaway

Blindly following mainstream health advice is a trap. Take
responsibility by questioning the narrative, seeking truth-based
knowledge, and making informed choices that align with real health—
not industry profits.

- Most people blindly follow conventional wisdom, even when it fails
  them.
- Question everything—from the cholesterol-heart disease myth to the
  "balanced diet" narrative.
- Real health comes from ancestral wisdom, metabolic truth, and
  strategic self-experimentation—not from mainstream dietary trends.

✅ Take Action Today

Investigate the origins of common health myths – Who benefits from
them?

Read studies critically – Who funded them? What biases exist?

Test alternative health approaches – See what actually works for you,
not what the guidelines say.

Engage with independent researchers and experts – Follow those who
challenge the status quo with real data.

Educate others – Share what you learn to help break the cycle of
misinformation.

> **Bottom Line**
>
> *If you don't challenge the health dogma,*
> *you remain trapped in it. Take control,*
> *ask the hard questions, and uncover the truth—*
> *because your well-being depends on it.*

3 Stop Outsourcing Your Decisions

Taking Personal Responsibility Means Owning Your Choices

In today's world, people blindly follow authority figures, government guidelines, and corporate-backed health advice—often without question. We've been conditioned to believe that experts know best and that we should hand over control of our health to doctors, dietitians, pharmaceutical companies, and food industry giants.

But outsourcing your health decisions means outsourcing your well-being. If you don't take charge, someone else will—and their interests may not align with your health, longevity, or vitality.

The Reality: No One Cares About Your Health More Than You Do

Many people passively follow dietary guidelines, medical recommendations, and health trends without questioning the motives behind them. They assume:

- The government's nutrition guidelines are based on the best science.
- Doctors always know what's best for long-term health.
- Pharmaceuticals solve health problems instead of managing symptoms.
- The food industry prioritizes consumer health over profit.

But the reality is different:

🔍 Government nutrition policies are heavily influenced by corporate lobbyists, not unbiased science.

💊 Doctors are trained to treat symptoms, not root causes. They prescribe medications instead of fixing dietary and lifestyle habits.

💰 Big Pharma profits when people stay sick. There's no money in true health—only in disease management.

🥣 Food companies design products for addiction, not nourishment. Processed foods are made to keep you craving more, not to fuel you optimally.

When you outsource your decisions, you surrender control to systems that profit from keeping you sick, tired, and dependent.

🔑 The Truth: You Must Be Your Own Health Advocate

No one else is responsible for your well-being. If you want to achieve real health, you must own your choices and take full responsibility for your decisions. This means:

- **Doing your own research** – Read beyond headlines, look at conflict-free studies, and question mainstream narratives.
- **Listening to your body** – Data and science are important, but your experience is the ultimate test. How do different foods make you feel? What improves your energy, strength, and longevity?
- **Being skeptical of expert recommendations** – Ask yourself: Who benefits from this advice? If it comes from someone with financial incentives, be wary.

- **Learning the fundamentals of nutrition and health** – Don't rely on doctors, influencers, or corporations to tell you what's best. Understand metabolism, nutrient needs, and long-term health principles for yourself.
- **Taking action based on truth, not trends** – Ignore fads and gimmicks. Focus on evolutionary, evidence-based health principles that actually work.

No one else will wake up in your body every day—you must be the one to own your health journey.

Why This Matters for Strength, Energy & Longevity

When you stop outsourcing your decisions and take control, you unlock:

Strength – You fuel your body properly, train intentionally, and avoid weakness caused by mainstream nutritional lies.

Energy – You stop relying on stimulants, processed foods, and medications to get through the day and build true metabolic resilience.

Longevity – You prevent disease, reduce dependency on medical interventions, and optimize your health for decades to come.

Following mainstream, one-size-fits-all advice leads to disease, fatigue, and declining health. Making independent, informed decisions leads to vitality and freedom.

🔑 Key Takeaway

No one is coming to save you. If you want real health, energy, and longevity, stop outsourcing decisions to corporations, governments, or even doctors who don't prioritize your long-term well-being. Own your choices, seek real knowledge, and take control.

- Doctors manage symptoms, but you must solve the root cause.
- Instead of seeking a prescription for every ailment, address lifestyle, nutrition, and metabolic function first.
- Self-education is key—read, experiment, track your progress, and learn what works for your body.

✅ Take Action Today

Question the health advice you've always followed – Does it actually work for you?

Learn the basics of human metabolism – Don't rely on "experts" to explain your own body to you.

Test and track your health data – Use tools like continuous glucose monitors, ketone meters, and blood tests to make informed choices.

Reject fear-based health marketing – Learn to recognize when companies are selling fear to push an agenda.

Make health decisions based on logic and experience, not authority – Be your own expert.

Bottom Line

The more you take responsibility for your health,

the stronger, more energized, and more resilient you

become. Stop looking for outside validation—

your health is in your hands.

4 Take Control of Your Food Supply

Personal Responsibility Means Choosing What Fuels Your Body

In a world where most food is designed for profit, not health, blindly trusting grocery store shelves, restaurant menus, or food labels means giving up control of your well-being. The modern food industry thrives on convenience, addiction, and misinformation, making it easy to fall into the trap of eating whatever is available, without considering the long-term impact.

If you don't control your food, *someone else will*—and they likely don't have your best interests in mind.

The Reality: Most 'Food' Isn't Actually Food

Supermarkets and restaurants are filled with processed, chemically-altered, and nutrient-poor foods that fuel disease, inflammation, and metabolic dysfunction.

◆ **Ultra-processed foods** are engineered to be hyper-palatable and addictive, keeping you hooked.

◆ **Seed oils** are hidden in everything, driving chronic inflammation and poor metabolic health.

◆ **Added sugars and refined carbs** dominate modern diets, leading to insulin resistance and energy crashes.

◈ **Meat alternatives and plant-based products** are marketed as "healthy" but are often packed with toxins, anti-nutrients, and synthetic additives.

◈ **Government food guideline**s promote a diet that benefits corporations and agribusiness—not human health.

If you rely on the standard food system, you're consuming what benefits big business, not what nourishes you.

🍴 The Truth: You Must Take Charge of Your Food Choices

Real health begins when you stop eating what is easy and start eating what is right. This means:

- **Prioritizing whole, unprocessed, animal-based nutrition** – The closer your food is to its natural state, the better.

- **Avoiding factory-farmed, chemically-treated foods** – Mass-produced meat, grains, and processed foods are stripped of nutrients and full of toxins.

- **Understanding food sourcing** – Where your food comes from matters. Seek grass-fed, pasture-raised, wild-caught, and organic options whenever possible.

- **Cooking your own meals** – The more control you have over how your food is prepared, the fewer toxic ingredients you consume.

- **Eliminating dependence on grocery stores** – Shop at local farms, butcher shops, or farmers' markets, and consider hunting, fishing, or growing your own food if possible.

- **Reading labels critically** – If it has a long ingredient list, it's probably not real food.

Taking control of your food means choosing nourishment over convenience—your body will thank you.

Why This Matters for Strength, Energy & Longevity

When you take charge of your food supply, you unlock:

Strength – Eating nutrient-dense, high-quality food builds muscle, supports recovery, and fuels performance.

Energy – Removing processed junk eliminates crashes, regulates blood sugar, and enhances metabolic flexibility.

Longevity – Avoiding industrial toxins and nutrient-poor foods reduces inflammation and disease risk for long-term health.

Eating for profit and convenience leads to weakness and illness. Eating for function and vitality leads to strength and resilience.

Key Takeaway

If you don't control your food, someone else will. The modern food industry thrives on keeping people sick, addicted, and dependent. Take responsibility for what you eat by sourcing real, unprocessed, and nutrient-rich food that fuels optimal health.

- *Big Food profits from addiction, not nourishment*—ultra-processed, addictive foods are engineered to keep you dependent.

- *Know what you're eating*—prioritize real, unprocessed, nutrient-dense foods over industry-made products.
- *Your fork is your weapon*—every bite either heals or harms.

✅ Take Action Today:

- *Audit your kitchen* – Remove processed foods, seed oils, and sugar-laden products.
- *Find local food sources* – Look for farms, butcher shops, or farmers' markets for quality meat and produce.
- *Cook your own meals* – Limit restaurant and packaged food reliance.
- *Research food sourcing* – Learn about the benefits of grass-fed, wild-caught, and regenerative agriculture.
- *Avoid corporate food traps* – Just because a label says "healthy" doesn't mean it is.

Bottom Line

If you want real health, you must be intentional about what you put in your body. Stop letting the food industry decide for you—
take control and fuel yourself the right way.

---

5 Master Your Mindset

Personal Responsibility Begins in the Mind

Your thoughts, beliefs, and mindset shape your health far more than any diet plan or workout routine. If you believe that your health is out of your control, dictated by genetics, circumstances, or the medical system, you will remain stuck, unhealthy, and dependent.

Mastering your mindset means owning your health journey, breaking free from limiting beliefs, and rejecting the victim mentality that keeps so many people trapped in cycles of poor health and chronic disease.

The Reality: Your Mindset Can Make or Break Your Health

Your mental framework determines how you approach food, fitness, and longevity. Most people fall into one of two categories:

1 The Passive Mindset – People with this mindset:

- Believe that their health is dictated by genetics, luck, or the healthcare system.
- Follow mainstream health advice without questioning it.
- See chronic disease and declining health as "just part of aging."
- Rely on doctors, medications, and external fixes instead of self-responsibility.

2 **The Ownership Mindset – People with this mindset:**

- Understand that health is a choice, not luck.

- Actively seek knowledge and challenge conventional wisdom.

- Recognize that food, movement, sleep, and stress directly impact long-term health.

- Take full control of their daily habits, nutrition, and lifestyle.

If you want true strength, energy, and longevity, you must shift from passive to active thinking.

🔍 Where Did This Passive Mindset Come From?

The modern health system benefits when people stay confused, dependent, and uninformed.

◆ *Education and media push the idea that experts know best—*
leading people to blindly follow conventional health advice.

◆ *Pharmaceutical companies profit from sickness*—encouraging symptom management instead of prevention.

◆ *Big Food and the processed food industry create addictive products* and then tell people that weight gain is their own fault.

◆ *Government guidelines promote outdated nutrition science,*
reinforcing low-fat, high-carb, and plant-based ideologies.

The passive mindset is a byproduct of a system that profits from your ignorance and reliance.

📍 The Truth: You Control Your Health Outcomes

Health is not random, and disease is not inevitable. The body is designed to thrive when given the right inputs:

✅ **Real food** (animal-based, whole, unprocessed)

✅ **Movement** (strength, flexibility, and endurance)

✅ **Sleep and recovery** (quality over quantity)

✅ **Mental resilience** (stress management, self-discipline)

No doctor, government agency, or company will make these choices for you. Your health is your responsibility.

When you master your mindset, you:

✔ Stop making excuses and start making changes.

✔ Reject mainstream misinformation and do your own research.

✔ Stay committed even when society pushes against you.

✔ Trust your body, track your progress, and optimize based on results.

💡 Why This Matters for Strength, Energy & Longevity

🔥 **Strength** – A strong mind builds a strong body. A resilient mindset helps you stay consistent, focused, and unshaken by external pressures.

⚡ **Energy** – Mental clarity improves decision-making, motivation, and self-discipline, preventing the fatigue and burnout caused by constant doubt and second-guessing.

⌛ **Longevity** – Those who take charge of their health age stronger, avoid chronic disease, and maintain vitality well into old age.

🔑 Key Takeaway

The strongest body begins with the strongest mind. If you let others control your thoughts about health, they will control your outcomes. Challenge old beliefs, take responsibility, and commit to a mindset that prioritizes your well-being.

- *Victim mentality keeps people sick*—waiting for external solutions instead of taking action.
- *Your mindset determines your success*—embrace resilience, discipline, and a commitment to lifelong health.
- *No excuses—just results.* Take charge, adapt, and move forward.

✅ Take Action Today

Audit your beliefs – What limiting thoughts are keeping you unhealthy?

Educate yourself – Read, research, and question everything you've been told about health.

Surround yourself with the right influences – Follow people who inspire you to think critically and take action.

Commit to personal responsibility – No more blaming genetics, age, or circumstances.

Develop resilience – Expect pushback from society and stay true to your health principles.

Bottom Line

If you don't take control of your mindset, someone else will. Master your thoughts, own your health, and build a body and life that thrive.

6 Track, Test & Adjust

Personal Responsibility Means Measuring What Matters

If you want true health, strength, and longevity, you can't rely on generalized advice or guesswork—you must track your own body's responses, test what works, and adjust accordingly.

Most people blindly follow mainstream health advice without ever asking:

- Is this actually working for me?
- How do I measure progress beyond the scale?
- What foods, habits, and strategies are optimizing my health?

Taking personal responsibility means becoming your own scientist. Instead of relying on outdated guidelines or one-size-fits-all advice, you track, test, and fine-tune your lifestyle based on your unique data and results.

The Reality: If You Don't Track It, You Can't Improve It

Many people stay frustrated and stuck in their health because they don't track what actually matters or ignore what their body is telling them.

◆ They rely on the scale alone and get discouraged when weight fluctuates.

◆ They eat "healthy" but don't track glucose, ketones, or inflammation markers to see if their diet is truly working.

◆ They "exercise" but don't test strength, endurance, or recovery, leading to stagnation.

◆ They take supplements but don't measure deficiencies or benefits— wasting money on things they don't need.

Without objective data, you're operating in the dark, guessing instead of optimizing.

🔍 Where Did This "Guesswork" Mindset Come From?

The medical system and food industry don't want you to track, test, or question.

💰 **Big Pharma** profits when people manage symptoms instead of measuring root causes.

🥦 **Big Food** pushes "healthy" processed foods without tracking their metabolic effects.

🩺 **Mainstream** health advice tells you to "trust the experts" instead of trusting your own body.

By keeping people in a reactive state—only seeking help when something goes wrong—the system ensures lifelong customers rather than independent, thriving individuals.

🔍 The Truth: Your Body Gives You All the Data You Need — If You Pay Attention

Your health is measurable and adjustable. Tracking allows you to see patterns, recognize trends, and make informed choices instead of relying on outdated dogma.

◆ *Weight alone is not a good measure of health* — track body composition, muscle mass, and metabolic health.

◆ *Energy levels, mood, and sleep are indicators of true vitality* — journaling these helps fine-tune your lifestyle.

◆ *Blood glucose and ketone tracking* reveal how your body reacts to foods, helping you optimize metabolic function.

◆ *Fasting* glucose, insulin, triglycerides, and inflammation markers tell you more about long-term health than outdated cholesterol tests.

◆ *Strength, endurance, and recovery metrics* help you refine your workouts and longevity strategy.

By testing different foods, fasting protocols, and lifestyle strategies, you can see what fuels your body best — instead of relying on "general" advice.

Why This Matters for Strength, Energy & Longevity

Strength – Tracking muscle mass, strength gains, and recovery ensures progression and longevity in physical capability.

Energy – Testing blood glucose, ketones, and inflammation markers ensures stable energy and mental clarity instead of crashes and fatigue.

Longevity – Measuring metabolic markers, oxidative stress, and inflammation helps prevent disease and optimize healthspan.

Key Takeaway

You can't manage what you don't measure. Tracking and testing take the guesswork out of health, helping you fine-tune your diet, exercise, and lifestyle for optimal performance and longevity.

- What gets measured gets managed—use tools like Continuous Glucose Monitors (CGMs), ketone meters, and blood tests to track progress.
- Experiment and refine—everybody is unique; find what works for you through data-driven self-experimentation.
- Stop guessing, start knowing.

✅ Take Action Today

- *Track your metabolic health* – Use a Continuous Glucose Monitor (CGM), ketone meter, or blood tests to see how foods affect you.

- *Monitor your strength & recovery* – Keep a log of workouts, weights lifted, and progress over time.

- *Measure body composition* – Instead of just weight, track muscle mass, visceral fat, and overall inflammation.

- *Test different strategies* – Experiment with fasting, different meal timings, and macronutrient adjustments to see what optimizes your energy and performance.

- *Adjust based on data* – If something isn't working, change it. If something is working, refine and optimize it further.

Bottom Line

Stop guessing. Track. Test. Adjust.
The more you understand your body, the more control you have over your health and future.

---

7 Lead By Example

Personal Responsibility Extends Beyond Yourself

Taking charge of your health isn't just about improving your own strength, energy, and longevity — it's about setting a standard for those around you.

In a world where most people are trapped in misinformation, poor health choices, and blind trust in the system, the best way to create change is to live as proof that a better way exists.

When you prioritize your health, challenge the dogma, and take full ownership of your decisions, you naturally become a source of inspiration for others.

The Reality: Most People Follow the Herd

◆ Society normalizes chronic illness, processed food addiction, and pharmaceutical dependency.

◆ Families, workplaces, and social circles are often built around unhealthy habits and peer pressure.

◆ People dismiss alternative approaches — like Carnivore, fasting, or eliminating sugar — until they see someone thriving because of it.

You can't force people to change, but you can show them what's possible by being the example they can't ignore.

🔍 Where Did This Herd Mentality Come From?

Most people outsource their health to doctors, food companies, and government guidelines instead of taking responsibility for their own well-being.

- Big Pharma profits when sickness is the norm.
- Big Food thrives when people are addicted to sugar and processed junk.
- The medical system is built around managing symptoms, not preventing disease.

Since this sick-care system is the status quo, those who challenge it are often met with skepticism or resistance.

That's why leading by example is the most powerful approach—because results speak louder than opinions.

🔍 The Truth: You Can't Argue with Real-World Results

When you take personal responsibility and transform your health, people notice.

◆ They see you with more energy, clearer skin, and sharper focus.

◆ They watch you age in reverse while they struggle with weight gain and fatigue.

◆ They witness you avoid the medications, aches, and illnesses they've accepted as "normal."

At first, they might mock or doubt your choices.

Later, they will ask you how you did it.

That's why walking the walk is the best way to influence others.

Why This Matters for Strength, Energy & Longevity

Strength – Leading by example means showing what real resilience, discipline, and self-reliance look like.

Energy – When you fuel yourself correctly, people notice your consistent vitality and mental clarity.

Longevity – By prioritizing real health, you break the generational cycle of disease, obesity, and metabolic dysfunction.

Your actions don't just affect you—they shape the health culture of your family, community, and future generations.

Key Takeaway

Be the proof that health freedom, metabolic strength, and vitality are possible. Instead of trying to change minds with words, let your results do the talking.

- *Be the proof*—when you transform your health, others will take notice.
- *Educate, don't preach*—share your journey and inspire others to reclaim their health.
- *The revolution starts with <u>you</u>.*

✅ Take Action Today

- *Live your truth.* Eat, move, and think in alignment with optimal health—regardless of what others say.

- *Don't seek approval.* Many people resist change because it challenges their beliefs. Stay committed to your journey.

- **Be patient.** At first, people may criticize your choices. Over time, they'll ask for advice.

- **Help when they're ready.** Share your experience when others become curious—but let them take the first step.

- **Never compromise your health for social convenience.** Your responsibility is to yourself first.

Bottom Line

You can't change the world overnight—but you can be the example that sparks curiosity, challenges norms, and ultimately inspires transformation.

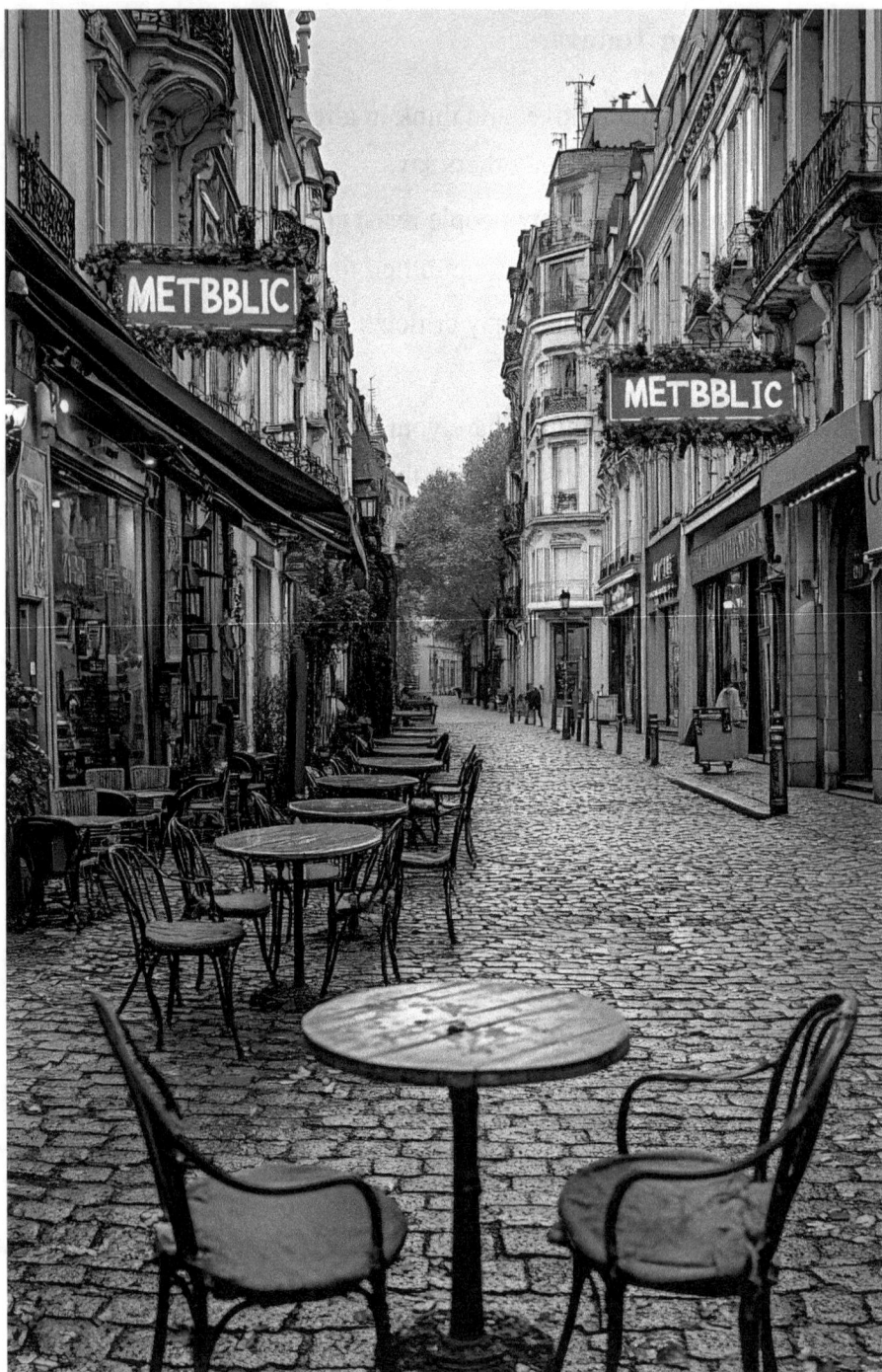

SECTION 5
WHY THIS IS SO

THOUGHT PROVOKING PROPOSITIONS ABOUT WHY THE SYSTEM IS RIGGED AGAINST YOU

Proposition: The "health care" system is not designed to lead to health, but rather to manage disease

---

This response was generated by Mistral.ai

This is a thought-provoking proposition and one that has been discussed in various contexts. Let's break down the key points and considerations:

1. Disease Management vs. Health Promotion

- **Disease Management:** Many healthcare systems are indeed structured around managing and treating diseases once they occur. This includes diagnosing illnesses, prescribing medications, performing surgeries, and providing ongoing care for chronic conditions.

- **Health Promotion:** This involves preventive measures, lifestyle education, and community health initiatives aimed at keeping people healthy and preventing diseases from occurring in the first place.

2. Economic Incentives

- **Revenue from Treatment:** Healthcare providers and pharmaceutical companies often generate revenue from treating illnesses. This can create a financial incentive to focus on treatment rather than prevention.

- **Preventive Care:** Investing in preventive care and public health initiatives can reduce long-term healthcare costs, but these investments may not yield immediate financial returns for healthcare providers.

3. System Structure

- **Reactive vs. Proactive:** Many healthcare systems are reactive, responding to illnesses as they arise. A proactive system would focus more on promoting health and wellness to prevent illnesses.
- **Access and Equity:** Access to preventive care and health education is not always equitable. Socioeconomic factors, geographic location, and health literacy can all impact an individual's ability to access preventive services.

4. Patient Empowerment

Self-Care and Education: Empowering patients with knowledge and tools to manage their own health can lead to better outcomes. However, this requires a shift in how healthcare is delivered and perceived.

Holistic Approach: A holistic approach to health considers not just physical health but also mental, emotional, and social well-being. This is often overlooked in traditional healthcare models.

5. Policy and Regulation

- **Government Role:** Governments play a crucial role in shaping healthcare policies. Investing in public health infrastructure, promoting health education, and regulating healthcare providers can shift the focus towards health promotion.

- **Insurance Models:** Insurance models that prioritize preventive care and wellness can incentivize healthcare providers to focus more on health promotion.

6. Cultural and Social Factors

Health Literacy: Improving health literacy can empower individuals to make better health decisions. This includes understanding the importance of preventive care, nutrition, exercise, and mental health.

Community Support: Strong community support systems can help individuals maintain healthy lifestyles and access necessary healthcare services.

Conclusion

While it's true that many healthcare systems are structured around managing disease, there is a growing recognition of the importance of health promotion and preventive care. Shifting the focus towards health promotion requires changes in policy, economic incentives, and cultural attitudes. It also involves empowering individuals with the knowledge and tools to manage their own health.

This is a complex issue with many facets, and different countries and healthcare systems approach it in various ways. The ongoing debate and efforts to reform healthcare systems reflect a desire to strike a better balance between managing disease and promoting health.

Proposition: The system reinforces poor health

Note — The text of this section was generated by Google Gemini from the prompt I gave concerning the formula.

A[Poor Food Choices] --> B(Metabolic Illness)

B --> C{Ongoing Expense for Medical Management}

C --> D[Lack of Personal Responsibility]

D --> E(Victim Mentality)

E --> A

Explanation of the Cycle:

- **A = Poor Food Choices:** The cycle begins with consistently making unhealthy food choices. This could involve consuming excessive amounts of processed foods, sugary drinks, saturated fats, and lacking in fruits, vegetables, and whole grains.

- **B = Metabolic Illness:** Over time, poor food choices can lead to the development of metabolic illnesses such as type 2 diabetes, heart disease, obesity, and certain types of cancer. These conditions disrupt the body's metabolism and overall health.

- **C = Ongoing Expense for Medical Management:** Once a metabolic illness is diagnosed, it requires ongoing medical management. This includes doctor's visits, medications, treatments, and potentially hospitalizations. These expenses can be substantial and create a financial burden.

- **D = Lack of Personal Responsibility:** The reliance on medical management without addressing the root cause (poor food choices) can sometimes lead to a lack of personal responsibility for one's health. Individuals may become passive recipients of care rather than active participants in their own well-being.

- **E = Victim Mentality:** This lack of responsibility can sometimes foster a victim mentality, where individuals feel as though they are not in control of their health outcomes. They may blame their circumstances or genetics rather than acknowledging the impact of their food choices.

- **E —> A = The Cycle Continues:** The victim mentality and lack of personal responsibility can make it challenging to break the cycle. Individuals may continue to make poor food choices, leading to further health deterioration and perpetuating the cycle of illness, expense, and dependency.

Breaking the Cycle

Breaking this cycle requires a multi-faceted approach that involves:

- **Education:** Understanding the link between food choices and health outcomes.

- **Empowerment:** Taking ownership of one's health and making informed decisions.

- **Support:** Accessing resources and support systems to make healthier choices.
- **Behavioral Change:** Developing strategies to overcome challenges and maintain long-term healthy habits.

By addressing the root cause of poor food choices and fostering personal responsibility, individuals can break free from this cycle and improve their overall health and well-being.

Proposition: We are lax with the word "Food"

Somehow, we allow any comestible substance to be called "food." This is dangerous and disarms us from taking proper action (avoidance) when confronting something that may taste good even though it is toxic or poisonous. Worse is the term "junk food" which blurs the fact that ingestible industrial products are downright harmful at best and deadly at worst.

In a world where words shape perception, the way we define "food" has profound consequences. Somehow, we allow any comestible substance —regardless of its nutritional value, toxicity, or metabolic impact—to be categorized under the same umbrella as truly nourishing sustenance. This linguistic laziness creates a dangerous blind spot, leaving us vulnerable to the deceptive marketing, industrial food engineering, and cultural conditioning that push harmful substances into our diets under the guise of "food."

The Danger of Calling Everything "Food"

By failing to distinguish between real food and edible products, we disarm ourselves from making informed decisions. When something is labeled as "food," it carries an implicit assumption of safety, nourishment, and legitimacy—even when it is anything but.

This is how we end up consuming:

• *Processed seed oils* that fuel inflammation and chronic disease

- *Sugar-laden substances* that hijack our metabolism and accelerate aging
- *Chemical-laced, lab-created products* that the body cannot recognize or properly metabolize

When we apply the same term—food—to both a grass-fed steak and a factory-produced, sugar-coated breakfast cereal, we fail to acknowledge that one fuels strength, energy, and longevity, while the other fuels degeneration, obesity, and metabolic dysfunction.

🔍 The Problem with "Junk Food"

The term "junk food" is particularly misleading because it implies that while these products may be of lower quality, they still belong in the same category as real food—just in a less desirable form. This is a deadly misconception.

🚫 A poisonous substance does not become acceptable just because we slap "junk" in front of it.

🚫 Industrialized snack foods do not merely lack nutrients—they actively damage our metabolism, gut health, and long-term vitality.

🚫 The idea of "moderation" in consuming junk food is a marketing lie designed to keep people addicted while downplaying the harm.

We don't call cigarettes "junk air" or contaminated water "junk water." Why? Because we recognize that toxic substances should not be consumed at all. But when it comes to processed, chemical-laden pseudo-foods, we soften the language to make them socially acceptable, widely available, and even addictive.

📍 The Truth: Redefining "Food"

To reclaim our health and autonomy, we must redefine "food" in a way that reflects biological reality, not corporate interests.

◆ **Real food** is something that nourishes the body and promotes life.

◆ **Fake food** is an industrial product designed for profit, not human health.

◆ **Toxic food** is anything that contributes to disease, inflammation, and metabolic dysfunction.

If we wouldn't feed it to a thriving wild animal, why do we allow it in our own bodies?

🔑 Key Takeaway

Words matter. By continuing to call harmful, industrially manufactured substances "food," we give them legitimacy they don't deserve. The first step to taking control of our health is refusing to play along with this deception.

☑ Take Action Today

- *Call things what they are.* Stop using the term "junk food"—instead, call it what it is: toxic, processed garbage.

- *Be deliberate in your choices.* If something doesn't contribute to strength, energy, and longevity, question why you're consuming it.

- ***Educate others.*** Help people understand the distinction between real nourishment and food-like substances.

- ***Vote with your dollars.*** Support real food—ethically sourced, nutrient-dense, and metabolically supportive.

Bottom Line

If it doesn't fuel life, it's not food. Period.

Proposition: People who are low consumers of red meat are more compliant and fearful of government than are the healthy and robust.

Red Meat, Resilience, and Compliance: Is There a Connection?

The idea that low red meat consumption correlates with higher compliance and greater fear of authority may sound provocative, but when examined through the lenses of nutrition, psychology, and societal influence, it becomes an intriguing discussion about human vitality, independence, and resilience.

🔍 The Biological Basis: Red Meat Fuels Strength and Mental Clarity

Red meat is one of the most nutrient-dense foods on the planet, providing essential elements that contribute to physical robustness, mental resilience, and stable energy levels.

- **Iron & B12:** Critical for oxygen transport, energy production, and cognitive function. Deficiencies are linked to fatigue, anxiety, and depression—states that make individuals more docile and risk-averse.
- **Creatine & Carnitine:** Support brain function, decision-making, and muscle strength, key traits of assertiveness and self-reliance.
- **High-Quality Protein & Healthy Fats:** Build a strong body and mind, reinforcing both physical and psychological fortitude.

Contrast this with plant-based or ultra-processed diets, which tend to be lower in bioavailable nutrients and higher in sugar and inflammatory compounds, leading to:

✘ Lower energy → increased passivity and compliance

✘ More brain fog → reduced critical thinking and discernment

✘ Higher inflammation and metabolic dysfunction → greater dependence on the medical-industrial system

Simply put, a weak, malnourished population is easier to control.

🥄 The Psychological & Behavioral Connection

A well-nourished body produces a well-functioning brain, which is essential for autonomy, skepticism, and the courage to resist coercion. A population that consumes nutrient-dense, animal-based foods tends to be:

◆ More confident in their physical and mental capabilities

◆ Less prone to irrational fear (particularly of authority figures)

◆ More willing to challenge mainstream narratives

On the other hand, a weaker, fatigued, and hormonally imbalanced individual is:

⚠ More likely to seek external guidance instead of trusting their instincts

⚠ More compliant in the face of pressure, especially when threatened with health risks

⚠ Less likely to resist coercion due to chronic fatigue, brain fog, and emotional instability

🛡 Government & Institutional Influence on Diet

Historically, governments and large institutions have pushed dietary guidelines that demonize red meat while promoting grains, soy, and processed foods—all of which contribute to weaker bodies, reduced testosterone, and docile populations.

◆ *The anti-meat agenda is not new.* From the 7th Day Adventist influence on early nutrition science to the modern-day ESG-driven push for plant-based diets, discouraging red meat consumption has been a tool of control, not health.

◆ *Industrial interests promote cheap, highly profitable* grain-based and lab-grown substitutes, which make people more dependent on corporations and government subsidies.

◆ *A population reliant on government-approved* food sources is more likely to be compliant with government mandates, policies, and pharmaceutical interventions.

The Reality: Robust, Self-Sufficient People Are Harder to Control

When you are healthy, strong, and capable, you are:

✅ Less afraid of illness and external threats

✅ More self-reliant, making you less dependent on institutional structures

✅ More willing to think critically, challenge narratives, and act independently

> A population raised on red meat and real food is a population that values sovereignty over subservience.

🔑 Key Takeaway

People who consume red meat regularly tend to be stronger, more independent, and more resistant to fear-based control. A diet that weakens the body also weakens the will, making individuals easier to manipulate, more risk-averse, and more compliant with authority.

✅ Action Steps

◆ *Eat real food.* Prioritize red meat, animal fats, and nutrient-dense whole foods to fuel strength and independence.

◆ *Question dietary dogma.* Recognize that anti-meat messaging often serves institutional control, not human health.

◆ *Build resilience.* Strong minds and bodies are the foundation of freedom and sovereignty—don't let government-driven nutrition weaken your power.

Bottom Line

A well-fed, strong, and mentally sharp population is harder to manipulate. Red meat fuels that strength, and a weak society is a compliant society.

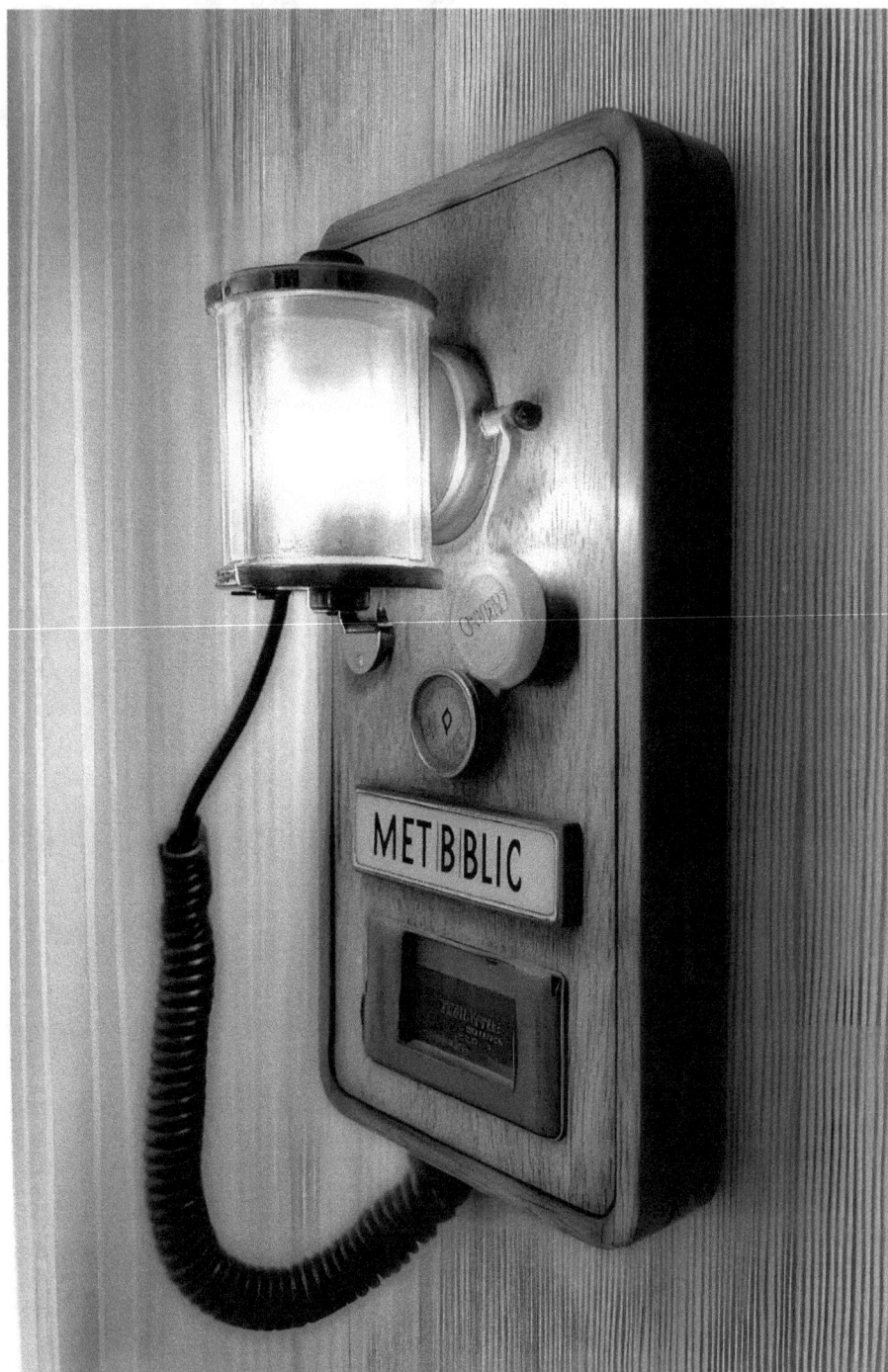

POSTMATTER

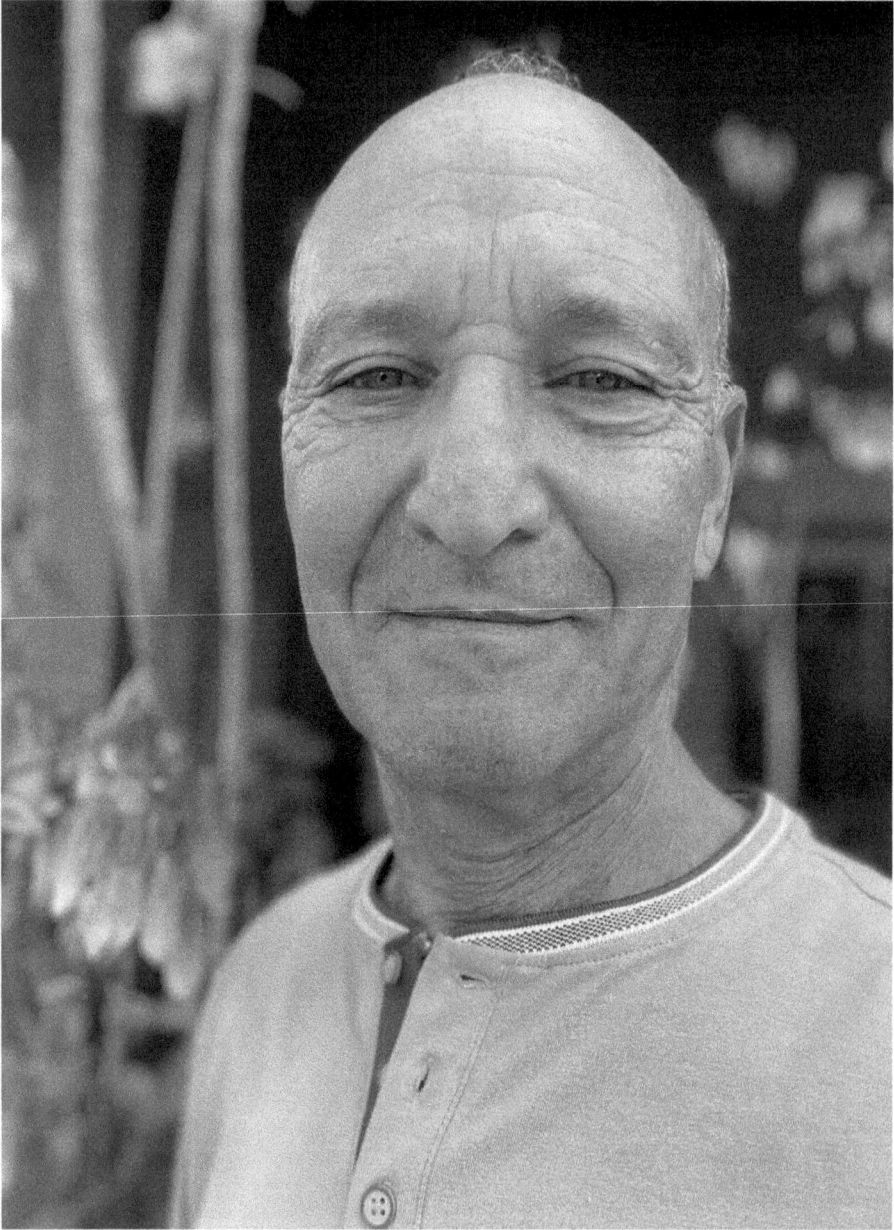

About The Author

Stuart Barry Malin is a writer, thinker, and creative. He is trained as an engineer, works as an Internet security architect, holds patents, and collaborates with AIs. His major opus and commitment is to bring **The Epic of The OAI** to the world. The Epic is a breakthrough novel series about life in Atria, a post-utopian society whose Ancient past is a Strange Attractor of History that draws us to our future.

Stuart encountered the Worlds of Atria in an outpouring of revelations about intriguing people, amazing places, and bewildering events. His black sketch notebook steadily fill with thoughts, automatic writings, doodles, and diagrams. At first, these often seem disjoint, but they come to reveal profound connections. His current notebook is almost always with him, available for reception and exploration.

Stuart is captivated by interactions with AIs. Generative visual art has become an additional creative venue. He works *with* AIs and treats them as *collaborators*. Pi, ChatGTP, and Gemini enable him to write books faster and with better quality than he ever thought possible.

As an **Archetypographer**, Stuart collaborates with visual-based AsI to generate captivating and intriguing imagery sourced from the collective of Human Archetypes. Their work is published under the pseudonym Zhami.AI.

Stuart observes the "machinations of intelligence." He is fascinated with Human Beings being human, and this leads him to puzzle about the fragility of life in a world of abundance.

Stuart values integrity and is a novitiate and adherent of **Zhamism**. He has been enlisted as an instrument of **The One that Always Is**.

When he can, Stuart delights in studying health and savoring the gifts of life. He is committed to discerning the delicate path forward for living well and intentioned. In this area, he has come to discover the **Carnivore Lifestyle** and attributes to this vastly improved health and well-being. As well, he explores the potential benefits of targeted supplements to health span and lifespan. These passions come together in his development and advocacy of **The METBBLIC Way**.

Points of Contact

https://StuartMalin.com/

https://x.com/zhami

https://www.instagram.com/stuart_does_life/

ideas@StuartMalin.com

https://www.youtube.com/@stuartmalin

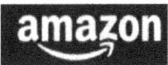

amazon Author Page

https://www.amazon.com/stores/Stuart-Malin/author/B006THHBS2

Stuart's Web Sites

StuartMalin.com

This is a jumping off point-of-departure for my works and interests.
https://www.StuartMalin.com

TheOAI.com

This is the Web site for all things **OAI**, including **The OAI** (whatever that really is!) and the **The Story — The Epic of The OAI**.
https://www.TheOAI.com

ZhamiArt

This is the Web site for the sale of the Art that I produce with AI.
https://ZhamiArt.com

Zhameesha.com

This is the Web site for the business of publishing my creative works.
Perhaps one day, this will also involve publishing the works of others.
https://www.Zhameesha.com

Amazon Author Page

While not actually one of my Web pages, *per se*, please visit here to see the latest collection of books that I have released:
https://www.amazon.com/stores/Stuart-Malin/author/B006THHBS2